Researching
Cultural Differences
in Health

Edited by

David Kelleher and Sheila Hillier

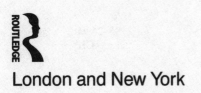

London and New York

First published 1996
by Routledge
11 New Fetter Lane, London EC4P 4EE

Simultaneously published in the USA and Canada
by Routledge
29 West 35th Street, New York, NY 10001

Routledge is an Independent Thomson Publishing company

Typeset in Times by
Datix International Limited, Bungay, Suffolk

Printed and bound in Great Britain by
Clays Ltd, St Ives plc

British Library Cataloguing in Publication Data
A catalogue record for this book is available from the British
Library

Library of Congress Cataloging in Publication Data
Researching cultural differences in health / edited by David
   Kelleher and Sheila Hillier.
        p.   cm.
   Includes bibliographical references and index.
   ISBN 0–415–11182–X. —
   ISBN (invalid) 0–415–11183–8 (pbk)
   1. Transcultural medical care—Great Britain.
2. Minorities—Medical care—Great Britain.
3. Minorities—Health and hygiene—Great Britain.
4. Health attitudes—Great Britain. 5. Health behaviour—
Great Britain.   I. Kelleher, David, 1935–   .
II. Hillier, S. M. (Sheila M.), 1944–   .
RA418.5.T73R47   1996
362.1′08′693—dc20   95–25980
                                                         CIP

ISBN 0–415–11182–X (hbk)
ISBN 0–415–11183–8 (pbk)

For our children

Charlotte, Clare and Ellen Kelleher
Katy, Charlotte, Ben and Martha Hillier

Contents

Tables

Contributors

David Kelleher is Reader in Sociology in the Department of Sociology and Applied Social Studies at London Guildhall University.

Sheila Hillier is Professor of Medical Sociology and Head of the Department of Human Sciences and Medical Ethics at the London Hospital Medical College.

Waqar Ahmad is Senior Lecturer and Head of the Research Unit on Ethnicity and Social Policy in the Department of Social and Economic Studies, University of Bradford.

Elizabeth Anwionu is Senior Lecturer in Community Genetic Counselling, Institute of Child Health, London.

David Armstrong is Reader in Sociology Applied to Medicine, UMDS.

Sharif Islam is a researcher in the Department of Dental Public Health at the London Hospital Medical College.

Helen Lambert is a lecturer in the Department of Public Health and Policy, London School of Hygiene and Tropical Medicine.

Myfanwy Morgan is reader in Sociology Applied to Medicine, UMDS.

Mary Pierce is Senior Lecturer in General Practice at Charing Cross and Westminster Medical School.

Suraiya Rahman is employed by the Education and Training Department of the London Borough of Haringey.

Leena Sevak is a Research Fellow in the Department of Epidemiology, London School of Hygiene and Tropical Medicine.

Chapter 1

Considering culture, ethnicity and the politics of health

Sheila Hillier and David Kelleher

> To cite 'culture' is merely to divert attention from the real objects of concern.
>
> (Francis 1993: 193; quoted in Smaje 1995)

> It seems incredible looking back, that while attention focused on the 'specific problems' of ethnic minority groups . . . an epidemic of coronary heart disease was sweeping the South Asian community and was the underlying cause of up to fifty percent of deaths. Why did this go unnoticed?
>
> (Bhopal 1993: 5; quoted in Smaje 1995)

Between them, these two quotations sum up the reasons why researching cultural differences in health may be regarded, at worst, as obscuring the impact of racism upon the health of minority ethnic communities and the health services available to them. At best, the activity could be regarded as an irrelevance, concentrating upon exotic difference or trivia. That ethnicity as an heuristic device for considering inequality or simply for the articulation of difference by which modes of domination or empowerment are produced under certain social conditions is a defensible research position is the theme of this book.

The 1991 census included a question about ethnic groups, and respondents were requested to describe themselves in terms of eight listed groups or to identify another to which they felt they belonged. The data is now beginning to be analysed and the collection of such statistics is justified on the grounds that this is a way of revealing the levels of socio-economic disadvantage from which ethnic groups suffer as well as presenting an overview of the health status of minority ethnic populations. The definitions of ethnicity were pragmatic, based on a mixture of skin colour, religion, national origin and self-definition, all of which are, at a common-sense level, deemed salient aspects of the classification of difference in contemporary Britain. Yet to many this is unsatisfactory, although often for opposing reasons. On the one hand, merely to draw attention, at an official level, to ethnic difference problematises ethnicity rather than focusing upon the racism which, it is argued, is the common experience of non-whites in Britain today. Another and contrary objection highlights the oversimplification of such categories as 'Indian', although it might be argued that these are an improvement on the use of 'Asian'. Such an objection seeks to increase difference in order to make categories representative of variety. It is obvious that any categorisation, however subtle, is, at best, an imperfect way of representing the reality of humankind. It is also clear that ethnicity is a shifting category which can change over time, whether defined by individuals themselves or by others. Therefore we must expect definitions to change and the relevance of some categories to increase or disappear, although current experience suggests that a proliferation of 'ethnicities' may well be the norm for the coming years. Whilst it is accepted that racism in social relations, which has a distinct class character, cannot be written off as 'failure to understand another's culture', this should not inhibit attempts to analyse cultural matters.

Government policies with regard to ethnicity and health policy have shown rather glacial movement over the last 30 years since the issue of 'immigrant' use of health services was first raised in 1965. Gradually, policies of assimilation have given way to an acknowledgement of pluralistic accommodation as now expressed in the Patient's Charter. This contains a specific emphasis on the need for awareness of and respect for 'religious and cultural beliefs', and recent writings in the health field display a willingness to take the issue of ethnicity seriously, together with the consequences for flexibility of provision that this entails. However, translating such intentions into practice lags far behind and displays all the difficulties of unclear goals and lack of appropriate knowledge and training that characterises the general relationship between research, policy and effective action. NHS reforms, which have put the burden of commissioning services responsive to Health of the Nation targets on localities, have brought the issue of dealing with both the special and the general health needs of ethnic minority groups into focus;

this immediately raises the question of patterns of utilisation, and the accessibility and appropriateness of ways of providing services. It has been suggested by a number of writers that so far the emphasis upon higher mortality rates (but fewer deaths) for diseases like TB (relative risk) has provided an inappropriate focus, that representation of members of ethnic minorities in health authorities is negligible, and the suspicion remains that patterns of socio-economic disadvantage will continue to be a major determinant of health outcomes, whether or not attention is paid to special or common needs within a framework of the understanding of ethnic characteristics.

In a recent comprehensive review of the available evidence, Smaje (1995) concluded that despite a wealth of literature on the health and health status of minority ethnic groups, patterns of health experience are inadequately described, let alone explained. It seems, therefore, far too early to close off the possibility that some aspects of minority health experience may be illuminated by considering values, beliefs, customs and lifestyles. That some of the work so far has been limited, dealing with stereotypes and occasionally patholo-gising minority cultures by assuming a majority norm, as suggested by a number of writers (Pearson 1983; Donovan 1986; Ahmad 1993), largely means it is bad social science, which does little to develop any understanding. Perhaps the point should be made, therefore, that most of the material has been produced within a biomedical framework, and an epidemiological one at that. Such a paradigm is not usually noted for the theoretical subtlety of its sociological categories. There seems room for a more complicated view of culture – that which is shared, believed and produced, as Rickword, stressing historical influences, suggests, 'the inherited so-lution to vital problems' (Rickword 1978: 103) or shared solutions to common problems. Ethnicity may or may not correspond with a particular culture. Sharing a culture does not imply merger between ethnic groups. Nor does common ethnic origin imply uniformity of culture. Therefore the two terms do not map directly onto each other. None the less, they are closely related. Brah has suggested that 'ethnicity emerges out of shared conditions – economic, politi-cal, cultural – to construct cultural narratives about these conditions which invoke notions of distinctive genealogies and particularities of historical experience' (Brah 1994: 812).

In the debates surrounding the value of such concepts as 'culture' and 'ethnicity' one is reminded of discussion a quarter of a century ago about the value of 'gender' as a category of analysis. It is difficult to imagine any piece of work which disregards gender today; but similar arguments occurred about the primacy of class over gender inequalities. In the event, 'gender' has proved durable throughout sociology, and has valorised methods and studies which emphasise the grounded experiences of the subject (Cook and Fonow 1990). Such studies continue to add to our understanding of health beliefs and experiences of and responses to illness (Cornwell 1984), which suggests that studies of relationships between culture, ethnicity and health are likely to be particularly successful and interesting when they lay emphasis upon the meanings and interpretations through which people make sense of their world. This material is most likely to be accessed by qualitative methods. This is not to suggest that there is no place for survey research or social epidemiology, but that the current imbalance needs to be addressed in researching cultural differences in health.

Most of the chapters in this book are case studies of health beliefs and behaviours in a variety of minority ethnic groups living in the United Kingdom – the majority in London. Although all chapters consider various methodological and theoretical issues raised by the studies which are reported, two chapters (those by Ahmad and Kelleher) take up these matters in greater detail, discussing points that have been raised in this chapter, and developing the arguments.

Ahmad argues that the volume of research on 'race' and health has not produced dividends either in terms of explaining differences in health experience or in improving provision to minority ethnic communities. He is critical of research that locates explanations for inequalities in health in ideas of cultural or biological pathology and which ignores the socio-political context. He considers the prospects for a more radicalised and empowering research agenda which will take into account the interplay of structural and cultural factors as elements of the context in which minority ethnic communities exist.

Kelleher's chapter deals with the complexity involved in disentangling material and cultural factors in minority ethnic groups and the difficulties surrounding the term 'ethnicity' itself, which is hard to define and whose subjects may change according to different context. He defends the idea of ethnic identity as an integrating concept for individuals, one which bestows a sense of belonging to a real or imagined community, psychological security and a range of goals. At a more practical level, he illustrates the importance of an understanding of attitudes and beliefs in providing appropriate health interventions. To this end, he advocates the use of ethnographic study and discusses the reasons for and against 'matching' researchers with the ethnic group that is the focus of the study.

The remaining seven chapters report a series of small-scale studies. The studies have a number of common themes or focuses. No less than three (Hillier and Rahman; Kelleher and Islam; Lambert and Sevak) are concerned to a greater or lesser degree with the Sylheti-speaking Bangladeshi population of Tower Hamlets. This group may rightly feel, as Hillier and Rahman report, that they have been somewhat overresearched without any notable improvement in health services. The dangers of exploiting ethnic populations for research purposes are ever present. In the research described by Hillier and Rahman it seemed clear that, where they existed, needs for advice and help with children's problems were not being met. Many people were unaware of services or were not referred on. In any case, they might be fearful of the close association between 'help' and the legal framework of child protection, as well as being less than wholehearted in their acceptance of the diagnoses of Western psychiatry. This chapter provides the raw material from which a more responsible service might be constructed, but it does not develop detailed recommendations.

Elizabeth Anionwu's work is also concerned with the acceptability of services. She reports the feelings of patients who are, among other things, research subjects for treatments of painful and unpredictable blood disorders. Since these disorders occur overwhelmingly in particular ethnic groups, she argues strongly that counsellors of a similar ethnic background to patients should be employed in explanations of treatment and in support. She describes a survey of counsellors, most of whom felt that ethnic origin was important in providing an appropriate service. There are practical implications to such a proposal, and Anionwu notes the lack of a counsellor capable of speaking any of the South Asian languages. The service she describes has now been set up in a number of UK cities, but still lacks the full complement of trained people.

The issue of 'matching' professionals and patients by ethnic group is also touched on by Hillier and Rahman, who note that referrals to the local child psychiatry service increased once Bengali and Bangladeshi professionals were employed. It remains unclear whether this was due to a greater willingness on the part of patients to be referred, or to the greater credibility with referrers which such employees conferred on the clinic. There is a strong suggestion in both Anionwu and Hillier and Rahman's chapters that, to be acceptable, services for ethnic minorities are likely to need to include members of those minorities. A different view, which is discussed by Kelleher, is the possible limitation of ethnic minority professionals/carers by directing them towards ethnic minority services. And it is self defeating and ethnocentric to argue that cultures are so impenetrable that only those born within them can understand their members. Acceptance of such a view would also render volumes such as this as valueless.

To take people's views of themselves either as individuals or as a group, their 'internal definition' of themselves, privileges the social resource aspects of ethnicity. The use of qualitative methods, as in most of these studies, where data is collected through face-to-face interviews, produces one version of social reality. It is important to remember, however, that ethnicity as a definition and the identification of cultural difference is something which is also done by outsiders. These same outsiders, in many cases the majority, have access to power and resources which may be denied to the group which is being defined and 'seen'; definition of others from the standpoint of power may have implications for how groups construct their identity. The conflict between ethnicity as resource and ethnicity as liability remains (Jenkins 1995).

Many of the chapters in this volume are concerned with the health beliefs of various ethnic groups and the impact of definitions of illness upon their daily lives. Morgan, and Pierce and Armstrong, in their studies of small samples of African-Caribbean patients, draw attention to the way hypertension and diabetes are defined and explained and to how dietary and activity restrictions are interpreted. Many of the views appear to be influenced by people's origins in the Caribbean, particularly concerning the use or dangers of certain foods and a general tendency to be sceptical of dietary advice bearing little relation to their own knowledge.

Lambert and Sevak make the important point that the often-observed 'cultural differences' can be exaggerated and that, when interviewed, Punjabi and Gujarati people show a wide range of views about the causation of illness. Certain themes emerge from all these accounts, however; worry, tension and stress, and the importance of hereditary and family history are all seen as relevant to health. The writers note that such explanations are characteristic of 'lay' health beliefs in general. In Morgan's chapter, the only one to compare the views of African-Caribbean and white patients, she notes that both groups regard stress or tension as the major cause of their ill health.

Religious belief as a way of dealing with and making sense of illness is discussed in a number of chapters (Hillier and Rahman; Lambert and Sevak; Kelleher and Islam). Belief in God and submission to God's will has sometimes led to misapprehensions for which the ethnocentric term 'fatalism' is used. These accounts make clear that illness or emotional disturbances are not passively accepted as being beyond individual control and that each person has a responsibility to look after their health and their God-given body. Lambert and Sevak make the point that intensity of religious belief may be found in many groups and that the pious in all groups may have more in common than less religious persons of the same ethnicity or religion.

Critics of cultural approaches to health, such as those cited at the beginning of this introduction, suggest that writers have focused on the marginal rather than the central health views of ethnic minorities, which in many cases resemble those of the majority. The blood disorders suffered by the patients in Anionwu's chapter are more likely to occur in ethnic minority groups, but no one could convincingly argue that to be concerned with them was merely a concern with 'exotic' health conditions. Indeed, the argument is the reverse: insufficient attention has been paid to these matters. Kelleher and Islam consider a group of Bangladeshi patients in Tower Hamlets. This group has a high prevalence of non-insulin-dependent diabetes. The group is also a Muslim community concerned to live by the laws of Islam. The study describes how it goes about the process of integrating the medical treatment regime with halal/haram distinctions and other cultural ideas about food.

Tower Hamlets is one of the few areas in the United Kingdom where there is a growing youthful population. The attitudes of Bangladeshi parents towards behavioural and emotional problems of their children are considered by Hillier and Rahman. Psychiatric services are among those most heavily criticised for racism in practice. In a speciality where individuals' own constructions of reality as well as the construction that others put on their behaviour are part of the matter under study, social and cultural settings are of great importance. But how are those to be understood? It is in the sphere of psychiatry that perhaps the greatest dangers exist for 'pathologising' culture, by failing to understand that the constructions and explanations which people put upon their behaviours are to be understood parenthetically. On the one hand, they must be seen against a background of migration, disadvantage and racism; on the other, as 'explanations-in-themselves'.

It is perhaps a point of criticism of this book that although most of these studies mention racism to some degree, there is surprisingly little mention of class. In some cases (Kelleher and Islam; Hillier and Rahman) this is because the populations are deemed to be fairly homogeneous in class terms. Although Lambert and Sevak draw attention to the fact that class differences may produce differences in health status, health beliefs and service utilisation in ethnic groups, the matter needs fuller investigation. Andrews and Jewson (1993) express dissatisfaction with current ethnic classification, arguing that it simply fails to reflect difference in a meaningful way and may obscure as much as it reveals, and the same applies to indicators of economic deprivation. It is clear that much more thought needs to be given to the important variables in any study that aims to avoid the 'empiricism of ethnicity' which categorises people in an unhelpful way. The salience of such variables to the community being studied must also be considered, including the notion that members may not classify themselves, or other ethnic groups, in the way that researchers do.

Andrews and Jewson suggest that greater refinement of ethnic categories, rather than simply relying on country of origin, may redraw ethnic boundaries 'along previously muted lines' (Andrews and Jewson 1993: 152). By the same token, the Irish remain hidden in the white population by virtue of their skin colour, although differentiated by country of origin. Kelleher and Hillier consider the fate of the Irish as an ethnic group and the patterns of health disadvantage which occur. In perhaps the most epidemiologically based account in the book, they consider the problems of second-generation Irish people and re-examine notions about Irish 'stoicism' in considering patterns of utilisation and psychiatric illness.

This book does not contain a unity of perspective. Despite similar themes, there are divergent views on the importance of cultural differences in health. Nevertheless, there is agreement that services should seek to be appropriate and acceptable, and a minimum requirement for this involves more tailored services, support of professionals from ethnic minorities and better attempts at communication, including listening. This approach should be accompanied by attention to cultural details. The dangers of 'lifestyle' explanations of ill health, which are given a cultural gloss in health promotion to ethnic minorities, are discussed in several chapters. The idea that cultures and ethnic groups are to be 'blamed' for producing ill health does not find any support in these pages. What is suggested is that people's meanings and needs can be better understood by listening to what they say about their own health. This applies to the majority as well as to minority ethnic groups.

Hall (1992: 259) defends the use of the term 'ethnicity' in words which might be seen as central to this book:

> the fact that this grounding of ethnicity in difference was deployed in the discourse of racism, as a means of disavowing the realities of racism and repression does not mean that we can permit the term to be permanently colonised . . . we are all ethnically located and our ethnic identities are crucial to our objective sense of who we are. But this is a recognition that this is not an ethncity which is doomed to survive, as Englishness was, only by marginalizing, dispossessing and displacing and forgetting other identities' . . . [It] is the politics of ethnicity predicated on difference and diversity.

It is in this spirit that we place before the reader a range of views in the debate, a series of lapidary studies and a number of methodological points and pitfalls which may be helpful to other researchers.

REFERENCES

Ahmad, W. U. (1993) *Race and Health in Contemporary Britain.* Buckingham: Open University Press.

Andrews, A. and Jewson, N. (1993) 'Ethnicity and infant deaths: the implications of recent statistical evidence', *Sociology of Health and Illness* 15 (2): 317–156.

Bhopal, R. (1993) 'The coronary heart disease epidemic in South Asians', *SHARE* newsletter 6: 4–5.

Brah, A. (1994) 'Time place and others: discourses of race, nation and ethnicity', *Sociology* 28 (3): 805–813.

Cook, J. A. and Fonow, M. M. (1990) 'Knowledge and women's interests: issues of epistemology and methodology in feminist social research' in J. McCarl Neilson (ed.) *Feminist Research Methods.* London: Westview Press.

Cornwell, J. (1984) *Hard-earned Lives: Accounts of Health and Illness in East London.* London: Tavistock.

Donovan, J. (1986) 'Ethnicity and health: a research review', *Social Science and Medicine* 19 (7): 663–670.

Francis, E. (1993) 'Psychiatric racism and social police: black people and the psychiatric services' in W. James and C. Harris (eds) *Inside Babylon: the Caribbean Diaspora in Britain*. London: Verso.

Hall, S. (1992) 'New ethnicities' in J. Donald and A. Rattansi (eds) *Race Culture and Difference*. London: Open University Press: 252–9.

Jenkins, R. (1995) 'Rethinking ethnicity', *Ethnic and Racial Studies* 17 (2): 197–224.

Pearson, M. (1983) *Ethnic Minority Health Studies: Friend or Foe?* Bradford: Centre for Ethnic Minority Health Studies.

Rickword, E. (1978) *Literature in Society: Essays and Opinions (II) 1931–1978*. Manchester: Carcanet.

Smaje, C. (1995) *Health, Race and Ethnicity: Making Sense of the Evidence*. London: King's Fund Institute.

Chapter 2

The meanings of high blood pressure among Afro-Caribbean and white patients*

Myfanwy Morgan

INTRODUCTION

The detection and treatment of essential hypertension, commonly referred to as high blood pressure, forms a major preventive strategy in reducing risks of cardiovascular disease. However, although the diagnosis of hypertension identifies an asymptomatic state whose significance lies purely in the relationship between blood pressure elevations and risks of coronary heart disease and stroke, people with this medical diagnosis may nevertheless undergo processes of adjustment to bearing a medical label which signifies their increased risk of cardiovascular events. Controlling blood pressure also often requires long-term drug therapy and attending regular blood pressure checks as well as reducing weight, modifying dietary intake and other lifestyle changes. The 'labelling' and treatment of high blood pressure thus imposes various costs on patients, including the need to cope with what Bury (1988) refers to as 'meaning as significance', in terms of the effects of the condition on the individual's sense of self and the reactions of others around them.

People's responses to a diagnosis of hypertension has formed the subject of a large number of social-epidemiological studies that have assessed the psychological and behavioural impact or outcomes of this medical 'label'. Studies of the 'labelling effects' of hypertension have been undertaken mainly in North America and are often associated with the introduction of worksite- and

* Afro-Caribbean has been used as a description of the respondents in this study as it is the term most widely used in the literature. The respondents had a variety of ways of describing themselves ranging from Jamaican to West Indian to Black Caribbean.

community-based screening programmes. Early studies undertaken at McMaster University based on hypertension screening programmes among employees at a steel foundry demonstrated an adverse impact of a diagnosis of hypertension on illness-related work absenteeism (Haynes *et al.* 1978; Taylor *et al.* 1981). This adoption of sick role behaviours appeared to be unrelated to whether the men were actually treated or to the achievement of blood pressure control, and suggested, therefore, that the labelling of this condition in itself had detrimental effects, thus raising questions about the personal, social and economic costs of this preventive strategy.

The findings of subsequent North American studies have mainly supported notions of an adverse labelling effect following a diagnosis of high blood pressure and have provided evidence of increased anxiety and lower ratings of psychological well-being, reductions in self-perceived health, or changes in work and social activities, although these effects were often reduced for patients who subsequently participated in and were compliant with treatment (for reviews see Macdonald *et al.* 1984, Alderman and Lamport 1990). However, a few studies, including research by Van Weel (1985) in the Netherlands and Kottke and colleagues (1987) in Finland have found no evidence of adverse labelling effects.

The British Medical Research Council (MRC) trial of mild to moderate hypertension also produced results which showed a positive effect of screening in terms of a reduction in the prevalence of psychiatric morbidity compared with baseline measurements among the trial entrants (compared with the control groups) (Mann 1977; 1981). This finding was mainly attributed to the positive effects for people with a non-psychotic disorder of the supportive relationships enjoyed through participating in the trial, and concerns were expressed regarding the effects on patients when the trial ended and the high level of support enjoyed was no longer provided. This positive effect of professional support accords with evidence that hypertensive patients participating in intensive treatment and follow-up programmes do not appear to exhibit the same adverse psychological and behavioural effects as patients treated by their usual sources of care (Polk *et al.* 1989). Such studies thus suggest that high levels of support from health professionals may exert a positive effect by influencing the meanings of this condition for patients. Also of importance in shaping the meanings for patients of high blood pressure is the influence of common images and patterns of belief prevalent in society that are conveyed by the media and by family and friends, including notions of the prevalence, causes and seriousness of the condition and of appropriate remedies. In addition, of significance at an individual level, is the influence of a person's own biography and circumstances, which consists of what Kleinman (1988) describes as an intimate type of meaning, in that aspects of the individual's life provide a framework within which ideas are assessed and evaluated. The process of 'making sense' of an illness, condition or medical diagnosis and assigning personal meanings therefore involves different sources of information and layers of interpretation and meaning which may overlap and interact.

Fitzpatrick (1984) thus describes patient-held ideas as 'syncretic' in origin, in that they derive from a variety of originally disparate and distinct sources and may be reworked and adjusted according to the concerns and experiences of individuals, with the result that it is difficult to disentangle the contribution of separate elements. He also notes that people's ideas may change over time in relation to new information, circumstances and experiences, rather than comprising a stable or fixed set of beliefs, while meanings may vary between societies and among different groups within a society reflecting differences in cultural values, expectations and experiences. For example, studies of Italians, Puerto Ricans and other ethnic minorities in the United States have demonstrated how their perceptions and responses to symptoms, the meanings ascribed to medical diagnoses and views of appropriate treatments, often differ in important ways from those of the general lay population (Harwood 1984). An understanding of the meanings of medical conditions for patients and the variations that may exist among different age, gender and ethnic groups in the population is thus crucial in promoting communication and ensuring that the information provided and decisions made by health professionals accord with people's needs and concerns.

Recognition of the significance of patients' beliefs and meanings for their adjustment and response to medical conditions has been associated with the development of this area as an important focus of research. However, the content of patients' beliefs and meanings regarding high blood pressure has received little attention, with the notable exception of Blumhagen's (1980) study of men attending a hypertension clinic in Seattle, which identified ways in which patients' beliefs about this condition differed from a formal medical model. Also, as several writers have recently noted, few studies in the UK have examined the content of patient-held beliefs and the meanings of medical conditions among different ethnic groups (Howlett, Ahmad and Murray 1992; Smaje 1995). Relating to this, the main impetus for the research described in this chapter arose from concerns expressed by a general practitioner regarding the difficulty he experienced in communicating with his Afro-Caribbean hypertensive patients and controlling their blood pressures effectively. This raised questions regarding the existence of cultural barriers arising from differences in cultural meanings and responses to this condition among Afro-Caribbean people compared with the general lay population. Moreover, the successful control of high blood pressure is regarded as of particular significance for the Afro-Caribbean community in the UK as, like their counterparts in the Caribbean, they experience a relatively high mortality rate from stroke, with SMRs for Caribbean-born men being 1.76 times the average for England and Wales and over twice as high for women (Balarajan 1991). There is also some evidence that Afro-Caribbean people and black populations generally have higher blood pressure levels than Europeans, which contributes to although not fully accounting for their higher incidence of stroke and higher mortality rates for this condition (Chaturvedi, McKeigue and Marmot 1993). However, the evidence is conflicting, with some UK studies not identifying any differences in the prevalence of hypertension between Afro-Caribbean and white populations (Smaje 1995).

People who classify themselves as black-Caribbean form the second-largest ethnic minority in England and Wales and comprised 0.9 per cent of the population in the 1991 census (approximately 500,000 people). Although people from the Caribbean have a long history of settlement in the UK, the largest migration occurred from the mid-1950s to the early 1960s. This was encouraged by the labour shortage and job opportunities during a period of reconstruction in Britain and made possible by the rights of citizenship accorded to Commonwealth citizens prior to the restrictions on immigration introduced in 1962. Afro-Caribbean people aged 40 years and over, who comprise the majority of hypertensive patients, thus consist mainly of people who grew up in the Caribbean and came to Britain as young adults during this period of large-scale migration. They may, therefore, be expected to have retained aspects of their traditional cultural beliefs, ways of thinking and behaviours. For example, in the health field there is evidence of the continued use of traditional herbal remedies among some sections of this original migrant group (Thorogood 1990). More generally, their explanations and meanings of diseases may be shaped by the survival and influence of medical belief systems, such as humoral theories, that are quite different from the scientific model, as well as being influenced by wider aspects of the culture, everyday lives and experiences of this ethnic collectivity (Dressler 1982).

The present research adopted a comparative approach and was based on groups of Afro-Caribbean and white hypertensive patients. This allowed assessments to be made of the extent to which patients from different cultural backgrounds share similar understandings and meanings of this condition, while recognising that the beliefs and meanings of high blood pressure among white patients may not necessarily accord with practitioners' perspectives. In view of the complex interaction and influence of ethnicity and socio-economic position, the study was limited to Afro-Caribbean and white patients from a working-class background, thus 'controlling' in this way for socio-economic position. However, although the two ethnic groups occupied a similar occupational position and socio-economic stratum, the Afro-Caribbean population nevertheless differed in their life situation as recent migrants and as a minority 'black' population within a predominately 'white' society. They may thus have experienced particular stresses and strains and problems of adjustment and discrimination as well as differing in what Giddens (1982) refers to as 'resources' or the structural properties which are drawn on (along with rules) by knowledgeable actors in the production of interaction. Gabe and Thorogood (1986), employing this notion of resources, demonstrated that differences in the availability, accessibility and acceptability of social supports, leisure activities, religion, housing, work and other resources between white and Afro-Caribbean women formed an important link between culture and structure, and served as enabling or constraining factors in managing illness and other aspects of everyday life. Thus, the meanings ascribed to medical conditions among different groups in the population and the responses they evoke may be viewed as products of differences in culture, life experiences and resources.

CONDUCTING THE RESEARCH

The research was based on groups of Afro-Caribbean and white patients who were being treated for high blood pressure by general practitioners in the inner London district of Lambeth. This district has the highest proportion of Afro-Caribbean people of any district in the UK. Thus, whereas people classified as Black-Caribbean formed the second-largest ethnic minority and comprised 0.9 per cent of the population of England and Wales in the 1991 census, they were the biggest ethnic minority group in Lambeth and comprised 12.6 per cent of the population (Teague 1993). Their residential concentration within areas of Lambeth also meant that Afro-Caribbean people comprised about 20 per cent of the patients registered with some general practices.

General practitioners at 15 practices in Lambeth were contacted and agreed to participate in the study. Six practices kept hypertension registers and in the other nine practices the general practitioners provided a list of their white and Afro-Caribbean hypertensive patients from which potential respondents were identified. The study group thus consisted of people diagnosed as hypertensive who had all remained in treatment, often over several years, and thus excluded what appear to be the fairly large numbers of people who drop out of treatment altogether (Hart 1987).

Patients were selected who met the following criteria: aged 35–55 (an upper age limit was introduced as one aspect of the research was to examine the impact of hypertension on work roles); diagnosed as hypertensive for at least one year to allow stable patterns to have developed; and not currently being treated for any other chronic condition. The frequent association of hypertension and diabetes among Afro-Caribbean people, together with the aim of selecting similar numbers of Afro-Caribbean and white patients from each practice, meant that large numbers of patients in the study practices were excluded from the group of potential respondents.

Of the hypertensive patients who met the selected criteria and who were in a manual occupational group 74 were approached for interview. No contact was made with nine of these people, three refused to be interviewed and two interviews were excluded as unsuitable. The final study group consisted of 30 Afro-Caribbean and 30 'white' respondents, equally divided between men and women. Initial contact was made through an introductory letter and followed up where possible with a phone call to arrange a time for interview. The interviews were conducted in people's homes and based around a schedule of questions developed through a series of open pilot interviews. This semi-structured approach aimed to focus on issues and areas of concern to the respondents, although the underlying framework of the study was researcher-generated rather than based on a community partnership model (Hatch *et al.* 1993).

The main study interviews covered aspects of patients' understandings of high blood pressure and its meaning in their lives, which forms the subject of this chapter, as well as issues relating to their use of the prescribed drugs and other remedies (Morgan and Watkins 1988; Morgan 1995). All interviews were tape recorded and generally lasted between 40 and 90 minutes. Content analysis was undertaken of the full interview transcripts and the original tapes were also listened to.

Interviews involve a social relationship between interviewer and respondent, if only for a short period of time. However, the nature of this relationship has an important influence on respondents' accounts in terms of the amount and type of information that is provided. Of particular significance is the influence of differences in ethnicity, gender and socio-economic background between the interviewers and respondents. Some interviews were undertaken by the author, who had a particular interest in the Afro-Caribbean population, having lived in Jamaica for several years, while the majority were undertaken by another middle-class female with experience of conducting semi-structured interviews. One group of respondents, for convenience referred to as 'white', were born in the UK, with the exception of three people who had come to England from the Irish Republic several years previously, and one from Spain. The Afro-Caribbean respondents were all born in the Caribbean, except two, who were born in Jamaica. They had come to Britain as young adults during the period of high levels of migration from the later 1950s to early 1960s, attracted by the job opportunities and especially the recruitment drives by London Transport, and had settled in south London. Most people were long-standing residents of Lambeth. Over half the Afro-Caribbean respondents and two-thirds of the white respondents had lived in Lambeth for 10 years or more and only three of the 60 respondents had lived there for under five years. Two-thirds of each group lived in council rented accommodation, consisting mainly of flats on large housing estates. Most of the other Afro-Caribbean people were owner-occupiers, whereas the other white respondents lived in private rented or housing association accommodation. Both ethnic groups shared a similar economic situation and comprised a relatively disadvantaged section of the population. One-quarter of the men in both groups were unemployed, and common occupations among the employed were caretaker, railway worker, general labourer and factory worker. Most women worked – the Afro-Caribbean women mainly full time and the white women mainly part time, with common jobs being clerical work, cleaning, cashiers and shop assistants.

The precise effects of the social characteristics of the interviewer on the nature of the relationship established with the respondents and the 'data' collected is difficult to determine. However, the interviewer felt well-received by all groups of respondents once initial personal contact had been made. People also appeared to be happy to talk about their 'blood pressure' and indeed often seemed to enjoy the opportunity to do so, subject to the general constraints of time and demands of other household members. However, the gender of the interviewers was associated with a reluctance to disclose problems of impotence. This is a well-known effect of anti-hypertensive drugs but was only mentioned by two men, and on each occasion when the tape recorder had been turned off.

The significance of differences between the race/class of the interviewer and respondents is likely to vary according to the nature of the topic and may be less important in relation to meanings and responses to illness (especially in relation to a non-stigmatising condition) than for topics with an explicit racial content or social desirability and prestige implications (Schaeffer 1980). The extent of cultural differences and shared meanings also varies between and within ethnic groups. In this respect it is notable that the Afro-Caribbean respondents had all been brought up in a culture that was strongly shaped by the white and predominately British colonial settlers and was characterised by a common language, dress, religious and educational system, as well as a common affinity with Britain as the 'mother' country (Goulbourne 1991). They had then spent over 20 years living and working in the London area in an ethnically mixed environment. Thus, as a group they are characterised by a high degree of integration and cultural assimilation, although they tend to continue to regard their own island or the 'West Indies' as 'home' and maintain aspects of their traditional culture, including aspects of diet and forms of worship and music. The culture of this sub-group of the Afro-Caribbean population thus forms a product of particular historical and structural processes and consists of an amalgam of their Afro-Caribbean traditions with the dominant values and institutions in Britain. A recent in-depth study of first- and second-generation Afro-Caribbean people indicated that the majority felt they had much in common with white British people, sharing common attitudes, aspirations and behaviour, although being aware of their non-acceptance as British by many white people (Modood, Beisham and Virdee 1994). This feeling of commonality on the part of Caribbean people with the white majority is likely to have been important in promoting a rapport and reducing the cultural/social distance between the interviewer and respondents.

In particular, it was notable that many Afro-Caribbean respondents disclosed in the interviews that they did not take the blood pressure tablets as prescribed, although they said they had not told their doctor about this. They were also willing to discuss their use of herbal remedies once they were aware that the interviewer was familiar with this Afro-Caribbean practice, and were often surprised at her knowledge about Caribbean herbal remedies which had been gained in the pilot interviews (Morgan and Watkins 1988). Thus, in these ways, they revealed their personal behaviours, rather than sticking to the relative security of what Cornwell (1989) refers to as a 'public account' or the reporting of behaviours that conform with their notions of a 'medical point of view' and expected behaviours. The differences in cultural background between the interviewers and respondents also meant that there could be fewer 'taken-for-granted assumptions', which probably often led to a greater emphasis on exploring and clarifying respondents' meanings. However, occasionally the interviewer felt reluctant to probe further, fearing that this might cause people to worry. This related particularly to the large numbers of Afro-Caribbean respondents who described how many of their relatives had experienced high blood pressure and died from a stroke, although, in contrast to the interviewer's own assumptions and interpretation, they appeared to derive comfort and reassurance from the 'normality' of their high blood pressure.

Cultural understandings and assumptions influence not only the dynamics of the interview and the data provided but also its interpretation. Recognising this, the themes and explanations developed in the process of content analysis were discussed informally with other Afro-Caribbean people as a means of checking whether the researchers' interpretation 'made sense' to them, thus providing a form of 'respondent validation'. However, a single interview can only begin to explore the complexities of meanings and behaviours among different social and cultural groups, and essentially serves as a starting point in promoting a greater awareness of the significance of ethnicity for patient-held meanings.

MEANINGS OF INITIAL DIAGNOSIS

A key stage in patients' experience of illness is the ascription of a medical diagnosis or 'labelling', which in the case of hypertension formally puts people in an 'at risk' category. For just over two-thirds of respondents this diagnosis had occurred during an ordinary general practice consultation, and especially when presenting symptoms of giddiness, dizziness, swollen ankles, tiredness or headaches. Other people had learnt of their high blood pressure during a routine medical check. For men this mainly involved a medical check undertaken for life assurance or work-related purposes, whereas for women problems of high blood pressure were more often identified in relation to the prescribing of contraceptive pills or during pregnancy.

There was a range of reactions to the initial diagnosis. A small group of people (four Afro-Caribbean and five white respondents) described themselves as feeling 'very worried', 'shattered' or 'very upset' on hearing that they had blood pressure problems. These people were all aged in their early forties or younger at the time and had learnt of their high blood pressure during a routine medical check. Their initial expressions of shock partly occurred because the diagnosis was so unexpected. These respondents also appeared all to have been aware of the significance of blood pressure in terms of the increased risks of a heart attack or stroke, with this awareness often being associated with the death of a close relative from these problems. This initial response of shock and fear is illustrated by the following people who, when asked how they felt when the doctor told them they had high blood pressure, explained:

'Bloody scared, for the simple reason being mother had high blood pressure and she died from a heart attack. That did frighten me. There was no pains, just this funny idea in my head that I was going to drop dead.'

(no. 61 – Afro-Caribbean respondent
diagnosed at medical check)

'Well, I was pretty upset because it does run in our family. Actually, my mother had it and obviously she died of a stroke at 76, so obviously that is all to do with hypertension.'

(no. 33 – White respondent
diagnosed at consultation for dizzy spell)

In contrast to these negative responses, the initial response to the diagnosis of high blood pressure was one of positive relief for four people (one Afro-Caribbean and three white respondents). These people had all consulted their general practitioner because they were worried about particular symptoms, and experienced a sense of relief on hearing that they had a rather lesser problem than they had feared. However, this initial relief was often tempered by subsequent concerns regarding the risks of a heart attack or stroke, as this respondent explained:

'I was relieved in a way to find out that I wasn't going mad, 'cos I'd got myself in such a state by this I thought I was going to have to go away [i.e., be admitted to a psychiatric hospital]. I didn't know exactly what was happening with me. I didn't mind until it sank in a little bit and then I thought, oh my God, blood pressure! It worries me a bit.'

[Why is this?]

'Well, because of heart attacks and strokes, that sort of thing.'

(no. 2 – consulted for feelings of giddiness)

Whereas small groups of respondents reacted in terms of either being shocked and upset or experiencing a sense of relief, for the majority of Afro-Caribbean (25 out of 30) and white (22 out of 30) respondents the initial diagnosis of high blood pressure did not cause them much worry or concern. A few people acknowledged that this was because at the time they did not really understand much about what high blood pressure was, nor did they realise its seriousness. However, for most people their lack of worry appeared to reflect the reassurance they received from the doctor that their blood pressure was not dangerously high and/or could be kept under control with tablets, as this respondent acknowledged:

'No, I wasn't worried. He [the doctor] gave me tablets and said they would keep it down a bit. No, I wasn't worried.'

(no. 54)

Although the possibility of controlling blood pressure with tablets and hence reducing risks often allayed concerns, many people added that they did not like the thought of having to take the tablets for the rest of their life.

Another factor which appeared to be important in reducing initial worry and anxieties among Afro-Caribbean patients was their perceptions of the 'normality' of the condition. Thus, they frequently cited other relatives with high blood pressure when explaining why they were not worried, and they appeared to derive reassurance from this. For example, one respondent, when asked if she felt worried when told she had high blood pressure, explained:

> 'No it didn't bother me much because you see my mum had it. It's in the family.'
> [So your mum had it?]
> 'Yes, my mum suffered with it until she died.'
> [How did she die?]
> 'A stroke, also my mum's sister and brother had it too. I've also had a brother that suffers from it and he's had strokes as well.'

> (no. 43)

Similarly, another respondent explained:

> 'It didn't worry me at all. You see, it runs in my family. My mum suffers with it and my brother. He had a stroke. He didn't know he had high blood pressure until he had a stroke.'

> (no. 35)

In response to further questions about whether she had asked the doctor why she had high blood pressure, this respondent commented, 'No, I just thought it was a natural thing. Some people get it and some people don't.' For some Afro-Caribbean respondents, the prevalence of hypertension and its familiarity thus appeared to reduce it's threatening nature, despite an awareness of the risks. It is unclear why a family history of high blood pressure and stroke may for some people reduce the level of upset and worry experienced whereas for other people it contributes to their worry. However, this may reflect differences in people's general orientation to life, both in terms of the importance attached to things being familiar and in terms of a readiness to accept one's fate.

The pattern which emerges is thus of a range of responses to the initial diagnosis of high blood pressure. Individual responses appeared to be influenced by both situational and personal factors. Situational factors included the circumstances in which the diagnosis was made, with feelings of 'shock' being most likely if this occurred during a routine medical check, and the experience of relief if they were consulting about symptoms which they feared were signs of a more serious condition. The doctor's reassurance concerning their blood pressure level and the possibilities of its control were also often important in reducing initial worries.

Personal characteristics influencing responses included people's awareness of the risks of high blood pressure, as well as their family history, which served either as a source of worry or provided reassurance.

LONGER-TERM MEANINGS AND RESPONSES

At the time of the interview all respondents had been diagnosed and treated for high blood pressure for at least one year and most for several years, and had therefore had time to develop their ideas and to acquire knowledge about this condition. Although the term 'blood pressure' was used in the interviews, respondents were asked if they had heard of the word 'hypertension' and if they knew what it meant. Only about half of both white and Afro-Caribbean respondents recognised that high blood pressure and hypertension were the same thing. About one-third of both ethnic groups said they did not know the meaning of hypertension at all, although most acknowledged that they had heard the term. Of the other 15 people, 11 respondents (one-sixth of sample) defined hypertension in terms of 'worry, stress or tension'. Further questioning indicated that 7 of these 11 people regarded high blood pressure and hypertension as distinct. Typical descriptions given by these seven respondents were:

'I've heard people say that they've got hypertension, which means that they're highly stressed. Nobody has ever spoken to me and said that I've got hypertension.'
[Have you ever heard of hypertension being linked with high blood pressure?]
'No, I don't see them linked together.'
(no. 19)

[Meaning of hypertension] 'Well, maybe that you are getting in a temper, you've lost your temper, that sort of thing.'
[Is this linked with blood pressure?]
'I don't think so, it's something different, getting in a temper and all worked up.'
(no. 26)

In contrast to this conception of hypertension and high blood pressure as distinct, the other four respondents described hypertension as something that could contribute to high blood pressure.

These people generally seemed to be concerned with the effects of hypertension in producing rises in blood pressure.

'I don't really know but I think it's [hypertension] to do with getting worked up which isn't any good for the pressure.'

(no. 15)

'Oh that's nervous problems or problems of the mind.'
[Do you see it as linked to high blood pressure?]
'Well it's the things that can bring it on and build it up.'

(no. 31)

There thus appeared to be a general lack of familiarity with the word 'hypertension' among this group of people, with only half being aware that it was another term for high blood pressure. The others either did not volunteer any definition or defined hypertension in terms of worry, stress and tension, with most regarding this as completely separate from high blood pressure. The pattern of responses was almost identical between Afro-Caribbean and white patients, with their lack of knowledge probably largely reflecting their general practitioner's reluctance to use and explain this term, preferring instead to talk about 'blood pressure'.

At the time of interview most respondents were aware that high blood pressure is associated with risks of stroke or heart disease, with all but three people naming at least one of these conditions. However, there was a difference between ethnic groups in the conditions identified. Altogether, 24 Afro-Caribbean respondents mentioned a stroke and only 18 mentioned heart disease (including 11 people who mentioned both conditions), whereas just 16 white respondents mentioned a stroke and 22 mentioned heart disease (including 7 people who mentioned both conditions). The greater identification of stroke as risk factor by Afro-Caribbean respondents accords with its greater prevalence among the Afro-Caribbean population. Similarly, heart disease was most likely to be mentioned by white male respondents, who have the highest rates of this condition. Differences in response between ethnic/gender groups thus reflected differences in their relative risks.

When asked about their current worries, 19 Afro-Caribbean and 13 white respondents said they did not worry at all. Other people acknowledged the fact that they worried at least occasionally, due mainly to fears of a heart attack or stroke and having had close relatives die of these conditions. People currently expressing worries had not necessarily felt particularly worried, shocked or upset at the time of the initial diagnosis, with responses to this situation differing from longer-term reactions. However, most people who acknowledged worrying also explained that this was not a continuous worry, but more something that 'occasionally crosses my mind', and 'sometimes you think about it'. These thoughts mainly occurred in response to specific triggers, such as collecting a new prescription, or experiencing feelings of tiredness, dizziness, pains in their chest or other problems that reminded them of their high blood pressure. A few people were also concerned about the wider social implications of this diagnosis in terms of its effects on their employment opportunities or life insurance, as this man explained:

'It bothers me at the moment because I'm job hunting and I have to put it down on the application form. I'm not sure how I would stand if I went for life assurance. Also there's lots of things that I would like to do but couldn't if it meant taking a medical.'

(no. 4)

Longer-term worries thus often appeared to be influenced by particular triggers and circumstances which shaped the meanings of their high blood pressure. The main reason given for not worrying or not being very worried was their belief that if they took the tablets and saw the doctor regularly then things would be all right, thus emphasising the influence of their faith in the doctor on the meanings of this condition. Several Afro-Caribbean respondents also again expressed notions about the 'normality' of the condition reducing their worries. Another feature of their responses was a tendency to acknowledge an acceptance of their 'fate', believing that 'when your number is up, then it's up'. As one Afro-Caribbean respondent commented:

'I take life as it comes. If that's the way I should pass off this world, then that's the way I will pass. I don't worry about death.'

(no. 29)

This apparent acceptance of one's fate conveyed by several Afro-Caribbean respondents may reflect differences in culturally shaped beliefs, possibly associated with the important place of religion in the lives of this generation of Afro-Caribbean people, and their familiarity during their younger years with a religious rather than a scientific ideology and set of beliefs. However, it may also reflect cultural differences in the expression of feelings, and thus identifies an aspect of patients' social reality that requires further study.

The more general finding that for most people their high blood pressure does not form a constant or continual worry was further confirmed by asking people whether there was any other condition they thought they might get. Less than a quarter of respondents identified any disease, of whom only six people mentioned a heart attack or stroke. The other seven respondents cited a broad array of conditions, which generally reflected their own past history or their family history and comprised pneumonia, bronchitis, cancer, Huntingdon's chorea and diabetes. Thus, although diagnosed as having high blood pressure and aware of its significance in terms of increased risks of a heart attack or stroke, only a small number of people felt at high personal risk of these conditions. Also, when asked if there was any disease they feared, no one mentioned a stroke or heart problems. The overwhelming response was cancer, which was mentioned by half the respondents, with only a few people mentioning any other conditions, which corresponds with Sontag's (1979) portrayal of cancer as the most feared and dreaded disease, a fear associated with the notions of the suffering it entails. A few people in the present study contrasted cancer with what they perceived as a fairly quick and therefore desirable death associated with heart trouble. The experience of living with or dying from a stroke was not mentioned, which may reflect the limited portrayal of this condition in the media and hence its lack of a strong social metaphor and meaning.

The diagnosis of high blood pressure thus often caused respondents to worry occasionally, but for most people it did not form a major long-term worry. This did not reflect an ignorance of the risks associated with high blood pressure but rather a lack of personal feelings of vulnerability, which was linked to their belief that their blood pressure could be effectively treated and was thus not a serious threat or, indeed, that it was currently under control. Such meanings are likely to have been influenced by both the information and reassurance conveyed by health professionals and by the wider meanings of high blood pressure and of the effectiveness of drug treatment within the lay culture. Also of importance in reducing worry, particularly among the Afro-Caribbean respondents, was an acceptance of their fate, while Afro-Caribbean respondents also appeared to regard high blood pressure as something fairly common and one of those things you might be expected to get, and as something thus 'normal' and understandable in these terms.

Given the fairly limited nature of the long-term psychological impact of hypertension among this group of respondents, it is not surprising that it had not caused many people to have changed their daily activities and social roles. For example, only five of the respondents reported changes in their work or time off work as a result of their high blood pressure. This group consisted of two men who had given up heavy labouring jobs because of their blood pressure, one station foreman who explained that he was not allowed to work if he did not feel well and was on medication, and two people who identified periods off work because of their blood pressure. No other changes in usual daily activities were reported as a result of their blood pressure problems, apart from a few people giving up jogging or sports because they thought this might be too strenuous and harmful. It is also possible that sexual activity was affected, although no information was given on this as a current problem.

Respondents did not think that their family members treated them any differently because of their blood pressure problems, apart from some of the men saying that their wives were careful about their diet. Indeed, people appeared to be surprised and even sometimes amused to be asked this question, and generally explained that their family did not regard their blood pressure as a problem since it did not affect their activities, and also they themselves rejected the notion that they were 'sick'. However, they often commented that they were not perfectly healthy because they had a medical problem and were being treated by the doctor. They therefore generally viewed themselves as not 'ill' nor quite 'healthy', but as somewhere in between.

Although people did not appear to have entered a sick role or to be regarded as sick by their families, an important effect of high blood pressure on their general life and activities was that they said they did not rush around as much and tried to relax and rest more and to avoid getting into arguments or getting 'worked up' about things. Indeed, when asked what they thought were the most important ways in which they could control their blood pressure, the most frequent responses were to rest, relax and avoid stress (mentioned by 17 Afro-Caribbean and 12 white people), to change their diet (mentioned by 11 Afro-Caribbean and 4 white people), and reduce weight (mentioned by 2 Afro-Caribbean and 9 white people).

Resting was identified not only as a general preventive strategy but also as a response to people's experience of physical symptoms, with about a quarter of each ethnic group commenting that they often felt tired, lacking in energy and needed to rest more. Thus, when asked about the effects of their blood pressure, this respondent explained:

> 'I just carry on as normal'
> [Have you changed what you do at all?]
> 'Oh yes, I do rest more. If I don't feel like going out I won't. I take things a little bit easier now. Instead of where I used to run about, I just stroll now.'
> [Why is that?]
> 'I seem to get more tired and need to rest. Also sometimes when I travel in a bus I feel sick. I don't know if it's my blood pressure or if my body is just like that.'
>
> (no. 38)

As this respondent indicates, although people often identified symptoms that they thought might be related to their blood pressure problem or its treatment, they frequently acknowledged that they could not be sure about the cause of these feelings and were aware that they might be due to ageing.

Whereas some people were unclear about the causes of their symptoms, others experienced symptoms which they interpreted as indicating that their blood pressure was 'high'. Altogether, two-thirds of the Afro-Caribbean respondents and half of the white respondents said that they were aware when their blood pressure was 'up', with the most common symptom being the experience of pains or 'sensations' in their forehead or sometimes at the back of the neck. This was often described as a 'pressure', 'fuzzy feeling' or being 'a bit like a headache but not quite', and was reported most often by Afro-Caribbean respondents. Other symptoms described were feeling weak or tired, problems of vision, dizziness or giddiness, awareness of their heart, feeling hot or feeling that their blood is hot. People's response to these symptoms was to rest for a while, and to take their tablets if these had been 'left off', as was common among the Afro-Caribbean respondents (Morgan and Watkins 1988). Confirming these findings, Meyer, Leventhal and Gutmann (1985) in a study of hypertensive patients attending clinics in Milwaukee, reported that 71 per cent of the newly treated group and 92 per cent of those who had continued in treatment for at least three months thought they could tell when their blood pressure was up,

with the most common symptoms again being a headache, awareness of their heart pounding and dizziness. Their respondents also
generally agreed with the statement that 'people cannot tell when
their blood pressure is up'. However, as in the present study, this
appeared to represent patients' formal knowledge rather than their
personal beliefs, and they frequently added such statements as, 'my
doctor tells me that people can't, but I can'.

Laboratory-based studies with regular individual feedback have
shown that patients can learn to predict their systolic blood pressure within 3 mm. Hg (Videgar, Lee and Goldman 1983; Pennebaker and Watson, 1988). However, Baumann and Leventhal (1985)
observe that there is no evidence that in an everyday setting, blood
pressure can be accurately monitored by patients nor of an association between symptoms and blood pressure, with the exception of
diastolic pressures over 130 mm. Hg. They thus believe that the emphasis placed by hypertensive patients on symptoms and the interpretation of symptoms as indicating that their blood pressure is up
may reflect their holding an acute symptom model of high blood
pressure which leads them to interpret everyday experiences, such
as normal physiological responses to high physical exertion, as
symptoms of high blood pressure.

Whereas resting was partly a response to general feelings of tiredness and fatigue and to people's perception of symptoms such as
headaches and dizziness, which they interpreted as indicating that
their blood pressure was 'up', this also formed part of a more
future-oriented preventive strategy, with respondents frequently
emphasising the importance of resting, relaxing and avoiding
stressful situations and tension as a way of controlling their blood
pressure. Thus, when asked what they thought were the most important ways of controlling their blood pressure, over half the Afro-
Caribbean respondents (17 out of 30) and just under half the white
respondents (12 out of 30) mentioned the importance of relaxing,
keeping calm and not rushing around. As this woman explained:

'Since I found I had blood pressure just over a year ago, I've
slowed down: I used to rush. I'm a terrible rusher for doing
things in the morning. I must have everything done, but then I
always try and sit down for a while if I know I've been rushing
and I would never have done that before. Now I would make
sure. I would try and sit down for a while and rest to try and
keep it down.'

(no. 15)

Similarly, two people who felt they could tell when their blood pressure was up explained their general approach to controlling their blood pressure in these terms:

'If I start to get worked up at work or even at home, it's not worth it. I try to relax.'
[So do you feel getting worked up is bad for your blood pressure?]
'Oh yes, definitely.'
[Do you just feel that, or has anyone told you?]
'I just feel that myself.'

(no. 62)

'I never think about it [blood pressure], just carry on a normal life. I try my best not to over do it. Don't get yourself overheated, over-emotional. These are the things that you are not supposed to do, because if you do that it goes up.'
[Who told you that?]
'Well sometimes I do find out myself.'

(no. 31)

These ways of managing and responding to their blood pressure emphasise the central role assigned by the respondents to relaxing and reducing stress and tension as a preventive measure and are associated with a general lay and patient-held view concerning the importance of stress, worry and tension as a cause of high blood pressure. Among the present group of respondents, stress, worry and tension was most frequently identified as a cause of their own high blood pressure and was mentioned by 13 of the 24 Afro-Caribbean respondents who were able to identify a cause of their own high blood pressure and by 14 of the 17 white respondents who identified a cause, whereas much smaller numbers mentioned conventional clinical risk factors of a family history of hypertension, being overweight and inappropriate diet (see Table 2.1). Blumhagen's (1980) study of men attending a hypertension clinic in Seattle showed a similar emphasis on stress and tension as the cause of their blood pressure problems and again his respondents assigned major importance to these factors in controlling their blood pressure. This led Blumhagen to identify the existence of two distinct models of hypertension, a medical model of 'hypertension' and a folk model of 'hyper-tension' with each conveying different meanings. However, although patients' emphasis on stress as a

Table 2.1 Patients' perceptions of the causes of their own high blood
pressure

	Afro-Caribbean (N = 30)	White (N = 30)
Tension, worry, stress	13	14
Familial, hereditary	4	3
Overweight	1	3
Diet	7	—
Smoking, alcohol	1	3
Other causes	2	2
Don't know[a]	6	13
No. identifying cause	24	17
Mean no. of causes reported	1.2	1.7

Note: Categories are not mutually exclusive
[a] These respondents were often aware of possible causes but did not think
they applied to them.

cause of high blood pressure contrasts with the professional
medical view presented in clinical texts, the possible influence of
psycho-social factors on risks of long-term elevations in blood
pressure, and not merely on short-term exacerbations, has formed
an important and continuing theme in the scientific literature
(Somers-Flanagan and Greenberg 1989) and includes recent
evidence from controlled trials on the positive effect of relaxation
on long-term blood pressure control (Patel *et al.* 1985). However,
the importance assigned by the lay population to stress and its
control is not confined to high blood pressure but also characterises
a range of other conditions whose precise etiology is unclear,
including cancer (Calnan 1987), arthritis (Williams 1986) and ill
health in general (Blaxter 1990). Some writers attribute this to the
increasing prevalence of social stress associated with the accelerated
pace of life and other features of modern industrial society, whereas
Pollock (1988) believes that it largely reflects the influence on lay
views of the elaboration and popularisation of the 'scientific'
concept of stress. As a result, stress may have come to be seen as if
it is something that occurs naturally in the world, thereby assuming
the status of a 'social fact', and as such it has direct implications
for the ways in which people perceive their world and make sense
of it.

CULTURAL MEANINGS OF HIGH BLOOD PRESSURE

Although the meanings of high blood pressure for patients often differed from formal medical views, there was considerable similarity in perceptions of this condition among the Afro-Caribbean and white respondents. This reflects the Afro-Caribbean respondents' length of residence in the UK, their common experiences of Western medicine and Western culture, and their similar socio-economic position to their white counterparts. Differences in patient-held meanings are thus likely to be greater for ethnic groups or subsections of ethnic minorities who do not share these common experiences.

Despite the general similarities in meanings across ethnic groups, there was some indication of a greater acceptance of high blood pressure among Afro-Caribbean patients as something 'normal' in terms of being very common and 'just one of those things'. This appeared to reflect their familiarity with blood pressure problems and their awareness of the condition's prevalence among black populations. In addition, although both groups placed considerable emphasis on worry, stress and tension as causes of their blood pressure problems, there was an indication that this was of particular significance to the Afro-Caribbean respondents. For example, they generally identified stress as the single cause of their high blood pressure, whereas the white respondents were more likely to identify more than one cause. Several white women also attributed their blood pressure problem to their own personality as being a 'born worrier' and 'living on my nerves', whereas Afro-Caribbean women all emphasised the effects of stresses and strains arising from difficulties and misfortunes of family members, problems of the disruption of family networks with relatives living in Jamaica, and housing and financial problems. The Afro-Caribbean respondents were also more likely to believe they could tell when their blood pressure was 'up' and rather larger numbers of Afro-Caribbean (17 out of 30) than white respondents (12 out of 30) identified relaxing and avoiding stress and tension as the most important ways of controlling their blood pressure.

There was thus some indication that a stress-related model may have been more widely and firmly held by the Afro-Caribbean respondents, although what was more important was the similarities in their beliefs and the meanings they assigned to their blood pressure problem, although they differed in their views regarding the appropriateness of long-term drug treatment (Morgan and Watkins 1988). There was also a greater emphasis among Afro-Caribbean respondents on the importance of diet in terms of eating healthy foods, defined as fresh rather than frozen, and including plenty of fruit and salads. These respondents were also aware that people from the Caribbean tend to eat too much salt and too much starchy food, such as yams, flour and rice, but, unlike their white counterparts, they rarely mentioned being overweight as a problem, with this difference in emphasis thus having implications for health promotion messages.

In broader terms, the diagnosis of high blood pressure, although often causing people to worry occasionally and to make some changes in their pace of life, did not appear to be associated with the severe adverse 'labelling' effects reported by many North American studies (Macdonald *et al.* 1984). This may partly reflect differences in the nature of the groups studied, including the relatively long length of time over which the present group of respondents had been under treatment, and the differences observed between the initial impact of the diagnosis and longer-term responses. However, differences may also exist between societies in the cultural meanings of this medical label and responses to health risks and medical diagnoses more generally. For example, a more aggressive approach has been taken to the detection of high blood pressure and to the thresholds for beginning drug treatment in the USA compared with the UK, as shown by differences in screening policies and in the blood pressure thresholds for treatment advocated by guidelines and consensus statements in the two countries (Joint National Committee, 1988; Swale *et al.* 1989). This difference in approaches to blood pressure control may be partly due to differences in health systems between the two countries, including the incentives for doctors to treat in a free-for-service system, the greater number of doctors in the USA, and the greater power exerted by drug companies in marketing their products. However, Payer (1989) suggests that the generally more aggressive approach to medical treatment in the USA also reflects a cultural belief in the possibility of exerting control over hostile elements, whether these are an inhospitable natural environment, extremes of weather, disease or other adverse circumstances. In this sense, the health system forms part of and reflects the broader cultural system. This accords with Parsons' (1972) description of the American value system as emphasising activism, worldliness and instrumentalism, and his belief that health is greatly valued in American society because it is an essential condition for another valued goal, that of achievement, which involves the imputed capacity to perform tasks and roles adequately. Thus, both medical professionals and patients may attach greater significance to the risks of blood pressure in the USA, with consequent implications for medical treatment thresholds, the information communicated to patients regarding the nature and seriousness of the condition, and the psychological and behavioural responses displayed by patients.

REFERENCES

Alderman, M. H. and Lamport, B. (1990) 'Labelling of hypertensives: a review of the data', *Journal of Clinical Epidemiology* 43 (2): 195–200.

Balarajan, R. (1991) 'Ethnic differences in mortality from ischaemic heart disease and cardiovascular disease in England and Wales', *British Medical Journal* 302: 560–564.

Baumann, B. and Leventhal, H. (1985) 'I can tell when my blood pressure is up, can't I?', *Health Psychology* 4 (3) : 203–218.

Blaxter, M. (1990) *Health and Lifestyles*. London: Tavistock.

Blumhagen, D. (1980) 'Hypertension: a folk illness with a medical name', *Culture, Medicine and Society* 4: 197–227.

Bury, M. (1988) 'Meanings at risk: the experience of arthritis' in R. Anderson and M. Bury (eds) *Living with Chronic Illness: The Experience of Patients and their Families*. London: Unwin Hyman.

Calnan, M. (1987) *Health and Illness: The Lay Perspective*. London: Tavistock.

Chaturvedi, N., McKeigue, P. M. and Marmot, M. (1993) 'Resting and ambulatory blood pressure in Afro-Caribbeans and Europeans', *Hypertension* 22 (1): 90–96.

Cornwell, J. (1989) *Hard-earned Lives: Accounts of Health and Illness from East London*. London: Tavistock.

Dressler, W. M. (1982) *Hypertension and Culture Change: Acculturation and Disease in the West Indies*. New York: Redgrave.

Fitzpatrick, R. (1984) 'Lay concepts of illness' in R. Fitzpatrick, J. Hinton, S. Newman, G. Scambler and J. Thompson (eds) *The Experience of Illness*. London: Tavistock.

Freidson, E. (1970) *Profession of Medicine*. New York: Dodd, Mead and Co.

Gabe, J. and Thorogood, N. (1986) 'Prescribed drug use and the management of everyday life: the experiences of black and white working-class women', *Sociological Review* 34: 737–772.

Giddens, A. (1982) *Profiles and Critiques in Social Theory*, London: Macmillan.

Goulbourne, H. (1991) *Ethnicity and Nationalism in Post-imperial Britain*, Cambridge: Cambridge University Press.

Hart, T. (1987) *Hypertension: Community Control of High Blood Pressure* (2nd edn). London: Churchill Livingstone.

Harwood, A. (1984) *Ethnicity and Health Care*. Cambridge, MA: Harvard University Press.

Hatch, J., Moss, N., Saran, A., Pressley-Cantrell, L. and Mallory C. (1993) 'Community research: partnership in black communities' in D. Rowley and H. Tosteson (eds) *Racial Differences in Pre-term Delivery: American Journal of Preventive Medicine*, supplement to vol. 9 (6), Oxford: Oxford University Press.

Haynes, R. B., Sackett, D. L., Taylor, D. W., Gibson, E. S. and Johnson, A. L. (1987) 'Increased absenteeism from work after detention and labelling of hypertensive patients', *New England Journal of Medicine* 299, 14: 741–745.

Howlett, B. C., Ahmad, W. I. U. and Murray, R. (1992) 'An exploration of White, Asian and Afro-Caribbean people's concepts of health and illness causation', *New Community* 18, 2: 281–292.

Jayaratnam, R. (1993) 'The need for cultural awareness' in A. Hopkins and V. Bahl (eds) *Access to Health Care for People from Black and Ethnic Minorities*. London: Royal College of Physicians of London.

Joint National Committee (1988) 'Report of the Joint National Committee on detection, evaluation and treatment of high blood pressure', *Archives of Internal Medicine* 148: 1023–1038.

Kleinman A. (1988) *Illness Narratives: Suffering, Healing, and the Human Condition*. New York: Basic Books.

Kottke, T. E., Tuomilehto, J., Nissinen, A., Enlund, H. and Piha, T. (1987) 'Hypertension treatment without labelling effects: the North Karelia Project', *Journal of Human Hypertension* 1: 185–194.

Macdonald, C. A., Sackett, D. L., Haynes, R. B. and Taylor, D. W. (1984) 'Labelling in Hypertension: A Review of the Behavioural and Psychological Consequences', *Journal of Chronic Disease* 37, 12: 933–942.

Mann, A. H. (1977) 'The psychological effect of a screening programme and clinical trial for hypertension upon the participants', *Psychological Medicine* 7: 431–438.

Mann, A. H. (1981) 'Factors affecting psychological state during one year on a hypertension trial', *Clinical and Investigative Medicine* 4: 197–200.

Meyer, D., Leventhal, H. and Gutmann, M. (1985) 'Common-sense models of illness: the example of hypertension', *Health Psychology* 4, 2: 115–135.

Modood, T., Beisham, S. and Virdee, S. (1994) *Changing Ethnic Identities*. London: Policy Studies Institute.

Morgan, M. (1995) 'The significance of ethnicity for health promotion: the use of anti-hypertensive drugs in inner London', *International Journal of Epidemiology* 24(3) supplement: 579–584.

Morgan, M. and Watkins, C. (1988) 'Managing hypertension: beliefs and responses among cultural groups', *Sociology of Health and Illness* 10: 561–578.

Parsons, T. (1972) 'Definitions of health and illness in the light of American values and social structure', in E. G. Jaco (ed.) *Patients, Physicians and Illness* (2nd edn). New York: The Free Press.

Patel, C., Marmot, M., Terry, D. J., Carruthers, M., Hunt, B. and Patel, M. (1985) 'Trial of relaxation in reducing coronary risk: four year follow-up', *British Medical Journal* 290: 1103–1106.

Payer, L. (1989) *Medicine and Culture: Notions of Health and Sickness.* London: Gollancz.

Pennebaker J. W. and Watson, D. (1988) 'Blood pressure estimation and beliefs among normotensives and hypertensives', *Health Psychology* 7 (4): 309–328.

Polk, B. F., Horton, C. C., Cooper, S. P., Stromer, M., Ignotius, J., Mill, H. and Blaszkowski, T. P. (1989) 'Disability days associated with detection and treatment in a hypertension control program', *American Journal of Epidemiology* 119 (1): 44–53.

Pollock, K. (1988) 'On the nature of social stress: Production of a modern mythology', *Social Science and Medicine* 26, 3: 381–392.

Schaeffer, N. C. (1980) 'Evaluating race of interviewer effects in a national survey', *Sociological Methods and Research* 8, 4: 400–419.

Smaje, C. (1995) *Health, Race and Ethnicity: Making Sense of the Evidence.* London: Kings Fund.

Somers-Flanagan, J. and Greenberg, R. P. (1989) 'Psychosocial variables and hypertension: a new look at an old controversy', *Journal of Nervous and Mental Diseases* 177, 1: 15–24.

Sontag, S. (1979) *Illness as Metaphor.* London: Allen Lane.

Swale, J. D., Ramsey, L. E., Coope, J. R., Pocock, S. J., Robertson, J. I. S., Sever, P. S. and Shaper A. G. (1989) 'Treating mild hypertension: agreement from the large trials. Report of the British Hypertension Working Party', *British Medical Journal* 298: 694–698.

Taylor, D. W., Haynes, R. B., Sackett, D. L. and Gibson, E. S. (1981) 'Long-term follow-up of absenteeism among working men following the detection and treatment of their hypertension', *Clinical Investigation and Medicine* 4: 173–177.

Teague, A. (1993) 'Ethnic group: first results from the 1991 Census', *Population Trends*, No 72. London: HMSO.

Thorogood, N. (1990) 'Caribbean home remedies and their importance for black women's health in Britain' in P. Abbott and G. Payne (eds) *New Directions in the Sociology of Health.* Bristol: The Falmer Press.

Van Wheel, C. (1985) 'Does labelling and treatment for hypertension increase illness behaviour?', *Family Practice* 2, 3: 147–150.

Videgar, L. J., Lee, R. M. and Goldman, M. S. (1983) 'Discrimination of systolic blood pressure', *Biofeedback and Self-regulation* 8: 45–61.

Williams, G. H. (1986) 'Lay beliefs about the causes of rheumatoid arthritis: their implications for rehabilitation', *International Journal of Rehabilitation Medicine* 8: 65–68.

APPENDIX

Table 2.2 Respondents by age and sex

Afro-Caribbean respondents			White respondents		
No.	Sex	Age	No.	Sex	Age
7	F	53	1	M	51
11	M	47	2	F	53
13	M	40	3	M	43
14	F	40	4	M	49
18	F	51	5	F	53
21	M	46	6	F	50
22	M	47	8	M	49
25	M	52	9	F	48
26	F	50	10	F	44
27	M	47	12	F	42
28	F	48	15	F	48
29	F	52	16	F	52
30	F	51	17	F	49
31	M	52	19	M	49
32	F	52	23	F	54
34	F	54	24	F	54
35	F	54	31	F	41
43	F	47	33	F	44
45	M	46	36	M	44
49	M	41	37	F	41
50	M	44	38	F	40
52	F	52	39	M	51
54	M	53	40	M	51
55	M	41	41	M	39
56	F	57	42	M	49
57	F	47	44	M	53
58	F	42	46	M	50
59	M	55	48	M	52
60	M	53	53	M	39
61	M	44	62	M	52

Chapter 3

Childhood development and behavioural and emotional problems as perceived by Bangladeshi parents in East London

Sheila Hillier and Suraiya Rahman

'No one else can do anything about these problems. If parents cannot discipline a child, who else can? These difficulties don't develop in a day. The child should have been disciplined from an early age. Doctors or medicines cannot help them.'

(A Bangladeshi mother from the community sample)

'I didn't want them to ask a child to draw and talk, these things are done in school. They should have checked his chest to see if there was anything physically wrong and x-rayed his brain. She [the therapist] wanted to see if he was using his senses – if he was mad or OK; that is why she asked him to draw things. I went for sickness – he was not eating, tearing his clothes and was not at peace.'

(Bangladeshi mother of a boy who had been referred to the Child and Family Consultation Service for slow learning)

The study reported here began as an attempt to answer a practical question. In 1990, clinicians at the Child and Family Consultation Service (Department of Child Psychiatry) of the Royal London Hospital wished to understand the reason for the apparently low consultation rates of Bangladeshi children. As the only available child psychiatric service within the London borough of Tower Hamlets in East London it was surprising that although 45 per cent of the children in the borough under 14 were described as being of the Bangladeshi ethnic minority they comprised about 7 per cent of referrals.

THE BACKGROUND

The extent of psychiatric morbidity

A number of explanations suggested themselves for the difference in referral rates between Bangladeshi and white children. Tower Hamlets is one of the two most deprived boroughs in a poor part of London. It could be that the number of white children referred with behavioural and emotional problems was abnormally high. No comparable morbidity or clinical data were available for services elsewhere. Another explanation might be that the existence of behavioural and psychiatric problems was actually lower among Bangladeshi children than the white population or any other ethnic group in the borough. Whilst there was no comparable data from Bangladesh which might provide a bench-mark, some research on South Asian children in Britain exists. Several authors have found a lower rate of child psychiatric problems, although they either did not include Bangladeshi children or lumped them together under the umbrella term 'Asian' (Kallarackal and Herbert 1976; Cochrane and Stopes-Roe 1977; Rutter and Giller 1983; Hackett, Hackett and Taylor 1991). An unpublished pilot study by one of the clinicians found that teachers in Tower Hamlets reported fewer psychological symptoms in Bangladeshi children than in their British peers (Marks 1994). The main differences lay in age groups across the whole sample, with older children showing more symptoms. A recent study (Newth and Corbett 1993) compared Birmingham-born children of Indian and Pakistani parents with white children and found no significant difference in the frequency of behavioural difficulties between the two groups.

The extent of psychiatric pathology in minority ethnic groups is a controversial area where a number of debates are played out. These include issues of reliability and measurement, definitions of ethnicity and the validity of psychiatric diagnosis, the role of racism or cultural conflict as etiological factors, and racist practice in psychiatry leading to the labelling of people as mentally ill. Questions as to the appropriateness of services are usually implicit rather than explicit.

Much of the data on the incidence of mental illness among ethnic groups is derived from hospital admissions (Cochrane and Bal 1989; Pilgrim and Rogers 1993). Hospital admissions are always a result of a number of social processes and represent how a particular set of behaviours has been construed by family members, members of the public, medical professionals or police. The high rate of African-Caribbean admissions for schizophrenia has been a focus of much attention and has been reported for several decades now (Bagley 1971; Littlewood 1992). Where the figures are seen as an artefact they have been variously attributed to inaccurate case definition, the possible 'drift' of the mentally ill to central or inner city districts where hospital admissions are more likely, and ethnic or cultural differences in the presentation of disease, resulting in minor symptoms being perceived as more serious by ethnocentric psychiatrists (Fernando 1991; Francis 1993). It has been noted that black doctors are less likely than white doctors to diagnose black patients inappropriately (Loring and Powell 1988). For those who accept that there may be elevated rates of schizophrenia in the African-Caribbean population, the explanation given is that pressures of migration (for older groups) and racism (for all ages), combined with low socio-economic status, are implicated.

As far as South Asian populations are concerned (Indian, Pakistani, Bangladeshi) the Cochrane and Bal study shows low admission rates relative to the general population (Cochrane and Bal 1989), although Smaje (1995), in an excellent review of the evidence, quotes several local small-scale studies where higher rates are identified. Much work took place before the 1991 census, so that the ethnic categories are not so clearly distinguished in early studies. However, the observation has been made that admission rates for Pakistani women are relatively low and it has been suggested that the diagnosis of schizophrenia or paranoia may lead to an 'exit' from the health care system. South Asian women show the highest rates of suicide and parasuicide (Balarajan and Raleigh 1993). When considering less dramatic forms of mental illness, researchers have found that the rates for GP consultation are lower, or similar to the rest of the population (McCormick and Rosenbaum 1990).

In summary, then, the available evidence raises more questions than it answers. Hospital admissions are only a partial guide to the incidence or prevalence of pathology. Mistakes in diagnosis may explain some of the figures, but the matter remains unresolved. In any case, far more attention has been paid to the issue of over-representation of ethnic minority groups, than that of under-representation.

The appropriateness of services: what do professionals know?

An earlier study from the same child psychiatry clinic in East London (Stern, Cottrell and Holmes 1990) noted that there was no difference between Bangladeshi and non-Bangladeshi children referred with regard to background demographic characteristics, presenting problem or attrition rates. Therefore, it would seem reasonable to conclude that Bangladeshi children were under-represented proportional to their presence in the local population. It is difficult for professionals to believe that there is not pathology 'out there' which is not being identified because of linguistic or service difficulties.

A note of warning must be sounded, however, against a stereo-typical view which occasionally surfaces – that of the 'passive' or 'timid' Asian, who, fearing stigmatisation or misunderstanding, will not seek help for mental problems when it is clearly in their best interests to do so. Hints of these approaches can be found, for example, in the suggestion that mental illness diagnoses are so stigmatising that they lead to a rapid 'exit' from the system. The reasons may be otherwise, and a possible alternative view is suggested below, which is related to the assessment made by ethnic groups about the effectiveness or appropriateness of the treatment on offer. Views of efficacy may also influence the process of seeking help in the first place, as many studies carried out on white British patients also show.

Stern, Cottrell and Holmes (1990) suggested that low referral rates at the Child and Family Consultation Service might reflect the fact that the clinic was failing in some way to meet the needs of the local population. In 1990, there were no Bangladeshi professionals working at the clinic. Later, a Bangladeshi interpreter and social worker joined the team. Finally, a Bengali psychiatrist was employed. A later study confirmed just how valuable such appointments were. In a survey of past patients in the clinic one woman said:

> If I could have used my own language I would have felt at ease. It would have been better for me to have a Bangladeshi professional, a Bangladeshi would have understood me. I could have expressed myself and the professional would have listened.
>
> (Hillier *et al.* 1994)

Furthermore, the attitudes of parents, GPs or schoolteachers to consultation and referral could have been influenced towards seeing little value in a clinic where they would have to rely on translation by family members. Few white professionals know even a basic greeting in Bengali. In Tower Hamlets, studies of Bangladeshi literacy have been undertaken which suggest that 80 per cent of fathers can read and write English compared with about 33 per cent of mothers, and 85 per cent of fathers can read and write in Bengali compared with 75 per cent of mothers (Tower Hamlets Education 1991). There have been no studies of fluency in English, however. More people may be defined as being unable to speak English than are able to understand spoken English. What this implies is that situations should be assessed carefully as to how far interpretation is necessary, either from family members or from hospital-based interpreters. The use of family members may cause difficulties within the 'family-oriented' consultation common in Western psychiatry:

> I tried to say things that my husband and daughter who were the interpreters, did not like. I wanted my daughter to be admitted to hospital, to find out why she wets the bed.
>
> (Hillier *et al.* 1994)

After the new appointments, increased referral rates from 1992 onwards were observed. Bangladeshi professionals were at least an insurance against gross misunderstandings and, at best, were able to share the meanings and concerns of the men and women who brought their children to the clinic.

The congruence between Bangladeshi parents' and therapists' definition of the problem from which the child suffered was an important determinant of satisfaction with treatment at the Child and Family Consultation Service (Hillier *et al.* 1994; Vanstraelen, Marks and Hillier 1996). This is an unsurprising finding, which perhaps would apply to any patient group, but it raises the issue of how far professionals' sensitivity should include cultural concerns. Fernando (1991) roundly accuses psychiatric professionals of having little or no interest in cultural issues. He attributes this to the mechanistic model which dominates Western psychiatry.

This model can be contrasted with the theory of mental illness used in Ayurvedic medicines, the traditional medical of India with which Unani medicine (an Islamic tradition practised alongside the Ayurvedic system in Pakistan and Bangladesh) is closely associated. Such a model distinguishes between mental illness caused by sorcery, that caused by the evil spirits or ghosts, and a disease described as 'malfunctioning of the head', often produced by shocks or setbacks in life (Bhattacharya 1986). Treatment for mental illness is not separated from bodily illness, and the tradition of introspection or a systematic theory of mind which characterises Western models of diagnosis and treatment is foreign to Ayurvedic thought. Of course, insanity is recognised and many of its symptoms are described. Pathological status derives not so much from behaviour itself as what is thought to be its cause. Therefore, syndromes would not necessarily exhibit the same range of symptoms, or symptoms would be described which are not observed in Western psychiatry. Kleinman (1987) has described the category fallacy which occurs in psychiatry when it attempts to impose categories derived in the West on the study of mental disorders in other cultures. Interestingly, the universality of Western categories is not extended to allow a similar universal status to syndromes which occur in other cultures.

It is important to recognise that different ideas about causation will not necessarily deter patients from seeking treatment eclectically and visiting Western psychiatric facilities as well as a local healer (see research report below) and also praying for the condition to be cured (Nichter 1981; Bhana 1986). In their evaluation of treatment, however, people may judge that the Western psychiatrist has simply not got to the heart of the problem. In our evaluation of the Child and Family Consultation Service (Hillier *et al.* 1994) one young girl was being treated by the clinic therapist for outbursts of anger or 'temper tantrums'. The parents judged that she had not been helped, and in fact was worse than before. They defined her illness as a persistent ear infection and remarked that she had 'red eyes' which did not get better. It was thought that the therapist had failed to attach any significance to the symptoms.

> They did not give us any medicine. They talked and asked us if things were getting better.
>
> (Hillier *et al.* 1994)

Unfortunately, this is sometimes interpreted by Westerners as inability to understand the 'talking cures' of Western psychiatry, together with an overreliance on physical treatments. The reality is far more complex. Discussion of emotional problems with family members or a religious healer is quite usual, but the mind/body distinction is not so rigidly applied. Therefore, in the case above, a cooling medicine can assist both the physical symptoms and the accompanying 'hot' behaviour/anger.

The understanding of alternative, culturally based models of mental illness, as Kleinman (1987) has advocated, may offer some useful insights into psychiatric practice. So far, such models have made little impact. Of less value are uninformed guesses at the cultural character of minority ethnic groups. For example: where mental pathology among South Asian groups is discussed, there is a tendency to leap to stereotypical conclusions about the 'Asian family'. If rates are low, this is attributed to the secure and stable environment provided by the 'Asian' extended family, which looks after members and relatives. As Parmar (1981) has pointed out, should some mental pathology occur, the same 'family' is castigated for its repressive attitudes, especially towards women, and its tendency towards physical punishment.

The inclination to pathologise cultures, about which a number of writers have complained (Pearson 1983; Ahmad 1993), is an ever-present danger which can only be remedied by better research, where definitions and lines of enquiry are made explicit and are accompanied by sensitive ethnography. In the clinic, practitioners may fail to recognise the racial pressures that can cause particular difficulties for individuals in the way they present themselves as patients. Reticence may be interpreted as deviant or 'secretive' behaviour; resilience as 'denial'. Misreading symptoms has been used as a partial explanation of the high rates of Afro-Caribbean schizophrenia, and one study has confirmed that diagnostic decisions are affected by the ethnic origin of the patient, with the cultural misreading that this implies (Loring and Powell 1988).

For many of the people interviewed in a recent North London study which included Indians, East African Asians and Bangladeshis, practical material problems were interwoven with emotional well-being (Beliappa 1991). Most of the people in the study said that there was a connection between how they felt about their socio-economic circumstances and symptoms such as lack of concentration, sleeplessness, excessive tension and feelings of nervous agitation. These data suggest that an ethnocentric construction of cultural issues, together with a lack of understanding of social and political circumstances, will be of limited value to patients. Practitioners who fail to take these matters into consideration will not be offering appropriate care and therefore will not be an attractive option for those suffering from mental problems.

One final matter which could influence parents in their attitude towards a child psychiatry service is the involvement of such services in the legal apparatus of the state. Consequently, the opinion of child psychiatrists is frequently sought in court cases, case conferences and situations where a child might be put into care. Agencies that have such powers are likely to be regarded by their potential clients with suspicion and fear. This is reflected in the remarks of one Bangladeshi mother who was interviewed for the study. She was commenting generally upon the issue of parental discipline:

'[Bangladeshi] parents in this country are very worried about the issue of disciplining children as they are fearful of them. As children know that they themselves can call the police if parents discipline them, this has developed fear among parents about their own children.'

Patient health beliefs, values, attitudes and knowledge

Littlewood and Lipsedge (1989) have argued that psychological abnormality will be recognised against a background of culturally produced repertoires of what is normal. Beliefs about normality and abnormality are therefore closely related and may, to an unknown extent, influence utilisation of mental health services. Understanding such beliefs illuminates the context of ethnic patterns of the utilisation of care. Some general information about health beliefs among white and minority ethnic groups emerges from the Health and Lifestyle Survey whose findings were analysed by Howlett, Ahmad and Murray (1992). The broad definition of 'ethnicity' almost confounds the findings; still the study shows that 'Asians' were more likely to view health in functional terms and to regard good health as a matter of luck.

Currer's study of Pathan women lends support to that view. She found that they were more concerned with the things that stopped them functioning, regarding unhappiness as something which they could not do very much about (Currer and Stacey 1991). Somewhat different is the work that has been done on 'somatisation'. This is described as the tendency to present physical symptoms which cannot be explained by 'Western' medical examination. It has been described as a means of presenting social and personal problems using a 'code' of bodily symptoms. It could be argued that the term 'somatisation' is misleading and ethnocentric. It suggests a level of unawareness in the patient, when the individual may be acutely aware of sadness and grief. Evidence for 'somatisation' comes from a study by Bal (1986), who found that patients interviewed after a visit to the GP did present psychological and social difficulties, using bodily complaints as a mode of communication that they thought would be more acceptable. Yet no greater tendency to somatisation has been found in other studies, or any that has was explained by social class differences (Bridges and Goldberg 1985; Bhatt, Thomenson and Benjamin 1989). The concentration upon somatisation should be seen as a reflection of the inflexibility of Western medical concepts and the rigidity of the body/mind distinction, rather than as 'inappropriate' presentation by distressed ethnic patients.

If patients are thought to 'somatise' their mental complaints, the view has also been expressed that they may be less likely to regard certain behaviours as symptoms of a mental disorder. This may be attributable to different ideas about the causes of mental disorder or to a wider tolerance of behaviours which Western psychiatry would identify as problematic. Newth and Corbett (1993) noted that Pakistani parents hold different expectations of their 3-year-old children compared with the white British population, and that they are tolerant of behaviour which British families might consider problematic. They were less likely to punish their children by smacking and more likely to distract them, using a toy or a sweet. The early work by Kallarackal and Herbert (1976) also suggested that certain types of behaviour were not recognised as problems by Indian parents. Newth and Corbett (1993) agree that behaviours were often seen as aspects of growing up, rather than problems or naughtiness. Although children's behaviour can cause distress to parents, they did not see it as a problem which required outside or expert help, nor as one that would respond to such help.

The three reasons invoked to explain apparent underutilisation of child psychiatric services – less need, less *perceived* need and inappropriate services – motivated the research team to investigate what a sample of local Bangladeshi parents might consider as normal or abnormal behaviour for their children, what they would do about it and what, if any, help they might seek. The study was carried out in 1992–1993.

THE RESEARCH STUDY OF BANGLADESHI ATTITUDES TO CHILD DEVELOPMENT

The Bangladeshi population in Bangladesh and London

Bangladesh, which came into existence following the Indo-Pakistan war in 1971, is one of the world's poorest nations. Its turbulent colonial history as part of the British Empire has contributed to many features of present-day Bangladesh, including its large population, its rural character and low level of modernisation.

The majority of the population are Muslim and the state language is Bengali. Of those Bangladeshis in Britain 95 per cent come from the Sylhet region and speak a particular dialect, Sylheti. The country is largely made up of the delta of three great rivers and the land is fissured with thousands of smaller rivers, creeks and streams, which makes fish a staple food. Most people participate in agriculture, but the land will not support the population and families often have to be engaged in a number of different industries, About 16 per cent of the population are landless labourers. In the countryside men are employed as boatmen and fishermen, car drivers, builders, potters, weavers, oil pressers, small traders or artisans.

Marriage is patrilocal. Women marry early and are expected to bear a son. Women play important roles in caring for the health of their family and making decisions about the use of health care, although they have less mobility than men and are expected to seek to achieve honour and respectability for their house by observing purdah. It has been suggested that the high degree of seclusion among Bangladeshi women, which is rare among the rural populations in Asia, regardless of religion, is popularly thought to be the result of attempts to protect them from foreign invaders (Abdullah and Zeidenstein 1982).

Because Bangladesh was part of a British dominion, Britain has been the country in which most Bangladeshis have settled (Adams 1994). Initial migration was of single men from small landowning families who took up employment as labourers in factories and in the clothing trade. The first settlers, who still retain their ties with Bangladesh in terms of land ownership, intended to make money abroad to enable them to buy more land at home. Most of the settlement took place in the 1950s and early 1960s. Strict immigration legislation in the 1960s and 1970s meant that men had to choose to bring over their wives and children or risk a permanent separation, so during this period and up to the early 1980s women and children from Bangladesh joined their husbands in the UK.

Tower Hamlets has the largest Bangladeshi community in the United Kingdom, comprising one-fifth of the total. They constitute the largest ethnic group in Tower Hamlets after the white population, comprising 23 per cent of the total population. Families are divided, with grandparents and siblings often remaining in Bangladesh while many younger children have been born and brought up in the UK, including a second generation of young Bangladeshi parents. There is, however, constant contact between families in Bangladesh and in the UK. Faster air travel and speedy methods of communication have assisted in maintaining ties between the two countries. Most of the members of this community are young. In Tower Hamlets 45 per cent are aged 14 and under and 40 per cent of primary school pupils and 25 per cent of the secondary school population came from Bangladesh. A small but increasing number of Bangladeshis are going on to higher education as the children get older. Most Bangladeshis are located in the west of Tower Hamlets, in Bethnal Green, Wapping and Stepney neighbourhoods, and a flourishing Sylheti community with shops, restaurants and mosques has grown up around the Whitechapel Road and the Royal London Hospital.

A number of studies of the health of the Bangladeshi population have been carried out and these suggest the male population have a higher than average incidence of heart attacks, diabetes and duodenal ulcers (Tunstall-Pedoe et al. 1975). The reasons for these patterns of ill health are not readily explained. It is commonly believed that the healthiest persons tend to migrate, and certainly overall mortality rates are lower than in the country of origin, however, from the point of view of those who must provide health services the prevalence of certain life-threatening conditions is of importance. (Marmot Adelstein and Bulusuo 1984). Whether or not there are particular environmental factors which have affected this population is almost uninvestigated. One early study looked at levels of smoking and dietary fat in Bangladeshi middle-aged men and recorded them as being at risk from heart attacks (Silman et al. 1985) but failed to consider issues of employment and environmental stress. There have also been a number of studies which have concentrated on the prevalence of diabetes (see Kelleher and Islam this volume). Bangladeshi men have the highest permanent sickness rates compared with all other ethnic groups in Tower Hamlets

(Banatavala and Jayaratnam 1995). Bangladeshi people are the least likely to have had contact with the preventive services. Less than 30 per cent say they feel well-informed about the range of health services available.

Social conditions in Tower Hamlets

Tower Hamlets together with its neighbour Hackney rank as the two most deprived boroughs in the country (ELCHA 1995). Most people who are in work have jobs as unskilled and semi-skilled workers. There are higher unemployment rates than in any other part of inner London. The total unemployment rate for Tower Hamlets is 22 per cent, but 46 per cent for Bangladeshis. Perhaps one of the most severe social problems in Tower Hamlets is poor housing. Local authority housing accounts for 60 per cent of housing in Tower Hamlets. Much of the housing stock is old and 10 per cent of council housing units are overcrowded. In the two wards with the greatest number of Bangladeshi families – Spitalfields and St Mary's – overcrowding runs at 28 per cent, and 50 per cent, respectively. One in five homes are unfit for habitation and 12,700 or more are unsatisfactory. The council house waiting list is 9,000, of whom 90 per cent are homeless and 80 per cent of those in bed and breakfast accommodation are Bangladeshi. It is clear that the Bangladeshis who migrate to Tower Hamlets are moving to a poor area.

It is not only material deprivation that is of concern but also the level of racial attacks and general levels of racism in the area. Phizacklea and Miles (1979) in their research in the inner city considered the way white racism is expressed. Crude stereotypes are certainly employed but racism also serves as part of the process whereby white residents attempt to make sense of public housing shortages, reduction in employment opportunities and other aspects of urban decline. In the eyes of many whites these matters were associated with the arrival of the migrant population who were thus blamed for the problems. Students regularly report racist abuse in schools and attacks are known about in the community, particularly one well-publicised case where a 17-year-old Bangladeshi spent six months in intensive care after being beaten up. The account that follows would seen to be fairly typical:

When I was in school every day was the same old day, I was getting involved in fights coming home with a black eye, being

called a Paki, having eggs thrown at your head at secondary
school. In school, out of school, walking down the street, getting
jumped at all the time because it was really bad 84-85-86-87. I
think those years were really bad, especially for people our age.

(Centre for Bangladeshi Studies 1994)

The role of Islam

The main mosque for the Bangladeshi community in Tower Hamlets is in Whitechapel Road and this is the focus of Friday prayers.
For Muslims Islam is part of life and regulates much of their daily
living. The community is generally regarded as pious. Many women
observe purdah in Tower Hamlets but many others do not and may
be seen walking to the schools and shopping in the major super-
markets with their children. Many are fully or partly veiled and
wearing traditional saris, part of which are used as covering for the
head.

Islam is a monotheistic religion which was born in the seventh
century with the revelations of the word of God to the prophet
Mohammed. These revelations were transcribed in the Qur'ān
and to these were added later sayings of the prophet which were
set down in the Habith or Books of Islamic Law. Together, they
provide a moral code touching on all aspects of the daily life of
Muslims.

Religious healing of the mentally ill in Bangladesh

Many people in rural parts of Bangladesh when they are facing
illness or distress initially seek help from religious healers. A large
number of villages in Sylhet are quite remote from hospitals and
qualified medical practitioners. Where faith is an integral part of
daily life and where every activity has a religious dimension, it is not
surprising that illness may not necessarily indicate immediate re-
course to medical help. Belief in God's kindness and concern for all,
in God's ability to protect suggests that He will, in the face of
illness, incline people to prayer to summon His aid. There is no
centrally operated health care system in Bangladesh and very few
hospitals in rural areas. Surgeries are run on a private basis and fees
are high, as is the cost of medicine, and this deters people who wish
to seek such help. Compared to allopathic (Western) medicine,
homeopathy is a cheap option. Herbal remedies have been used

traditionally by rural people and about 70 per cent of illness is treated thus.

At present there are no facilities available in hospitals or the established medical colleges to deal with the emotional problems of children in Bangladesh. In rural areas it is the close-knit families which provide support and comfort in distress. One study explored perceptions of mental illness and its causation in a rural community in South India (Srinivasa and Trivedi 1982). It found that there was a clear concept of madness which was identified by mood changes, violent behaviour and sleep disturbance. Such illnesses could be attributed to extraneous forces such as evil spirits, a curse, germs, financial worries or to intrinsic factors such as brain disorder or sudden trauma. The majority of those surveyed in that study suggested a mixture of extraneous intrinsic factors attributing illness to mental worries or a curse. The similarity with ideas of mental illness causation in Bangladesh described by Bhattacharya is clear. *Paglami* or madness can be composed of different elements, that is, *bhuta bhara* (ghost possession), *tukataka* (sorcery, a curse) and *mathhar golmal* (disease of the head), which can be brought on by traumatic shock. Bengalis use the term *upri* to describe extraneous and non-physical forces which can also be called *bhuta*, implying the involvement of a jinnee or ghost. For example, the spirit of someone who has died in unfortunate circumstances can exert an evil influence. The signs of the influence of *upri* are excessive fear in a child, many bad dreams, bed wetting in teenagers, a tendency of a child to change colour, refusal of breast milk by a very young child, talking in one's sleep. For such illnesses a religious healer, a mullah, would be chosen to help and would be the first point of call. The mullah's prayers would be calming and reassuring. He might also read Qur'ānic verses, perform a 'blow' (a gentle breath of air over the person) or provide *taviz* (Qur'ānic verses enclosed in an amulet) and a spiritual talisman to ward off the evil influences. However, those patients who believe in supernatural causation of illness will also seek and accept parallel modes of treatment believing both to be of value.

A family may also consult a hakim, the traditional healer in Bangladesh who is a scholar with learning and wisdom. Usually a Unani practitioner, he treats diseases with traditional herbal remedies but also takes into account the familial, social and religious context of the patient. A hakim with knowledge of the family provides counsel about losses and stresses they have experienced and thus provides effective treatment for anxieties and somatic complaints arising from stress in much the same way as a Western therapist working with a psychodynamic model.

Hakims practice in the UK and may well be the first source of help for what may be identified as minor illnesses. Consultation with religious healers is probably quite widespread, and the study below gives evidence of this, although respondents were sometimes reluctant to talk extensively about it. However, one woman said:

'I had acute pain in my chest and stomach, medical treatments could not cure them. I was cured by my own treatment. The recitation of a verse from the Qur'ān [*Sura Yasim*] helped me to recover. I do not have the pain anymore.'

Child psychiatry in Britain

Child psychiatry in Britain uses a number of theories eclectically. From developmental psychology, it takes the notion of appropriate growth and development. The object relations school furnishes a model of family functioning. The therapeutic paradigm is broadly psychodynamic, therefore treatments tend to use psychotherapy and behavioural or cognitive therapies. There is relatively little reliance on a drug regime, in contrast to adult psychiatry. Child psychiatry deals with a very wide range of problems. These may include the behavioural side-effects of physical problems like epilepsy or cerebal palsy as well as the physical symptoms which are believed to result from psychological disturbance, for example, enuresis and enco-presis or hyperactivity. Speech delays, educational difficulties, such as limited literacy skills or non attendance at school, and learning difficulties are also included. Failure to eat, telling lies, aggressive violent behaviour with siblings or at school, solvent abuse, temper tantrums and self-injury, head banging, breathing problems and self-mutilitation are disorders with which child psychiatrists deal. Finally, physical and sexual abuse is brought to their attention.

Clearly, many of these symptoms and syndromes are related to the social context in which the child lives. For example, school phobia would not be possible in a country where children do not routinely attend school. So there is a certain amount of cultural boundedness in those matters with which child psychiatry deals and this is an important problem when considering the uptake of services by another ethnic group.

Are the norms and standards of behaviour which are regarded in Western psychiatry and Western society as appropriate for children shared by the ethnic group? If not, there would be reasonable grounds for finding out what their norms and standards are and how they may differ, and from these to understand what they do regard as behavioural and emotional difficulties of children. On the recognition of such behavioural difficulties, what do parents feel is an appropriate way of dealing with them? These were the research questions which were developed.

Methodology: The questionnaire, the researcher and the sample

A semi-structured questionnaire was used. It concentrated on looking at expectations of development for children of particular ages, bearing in mind that our sample would cover both young and adolescent children. The questionnaire, which was translated and back-translated into and from Bengali, covered the following areas:

Demographic background   This gave information about the number of children, their ages, and employment of the adult members of the household.

Social support   There was an attempt to establish the level of social support which each woman enjoyed. They were questioned about whom they went to when they had a problem and how frequently they visited members of their own or their husband's family who lived outside the household. These responses were combined to provide an index of social support which was then correlated with the identification of worrying behaviours in children. The hypothesis was that the lower the level of social support the greater the tendency to identify behaviours in children as worrying.

Religious observance   This dealt with the respondent's religious background and asked them about their religious observances, the time they had for praying and fasting, the degree to which they encouraged children to have extra Arabic lessons and any difficulties they had in keeping up their religious observances. They were also asked to contrast their own upbringing with that of their children.

Child development   The questionnaire then moved on to children's developmental stages and was heavily influenced by child psychiatric concepts. The questionnaire asked about the tasks expected of boys and girls at ages 4, 8 and 15. The questionnaire also covered issues of bowel control and when a child would be expected to be dry.

Help seeking   Parents were asked to comment upon what they thought would be naughty behaviour, how they would discipline a child, what aspect of children's behaviour would worry them. Parents were also asked what they would do if a child persisted in behaviour of which they did not approve. They were also asked about how they coped with a child's illness, naughtiness or unhappiness in Bangladesh or England, and where they went for help.

Cinical vignettes   Finally, mothers were presented with two clinical vignettes, one for girls aged 15 and one for boys aged 15, and asked in detail about what help they would expect and to whom they would go for advice. An open-ended questionnaire of this sort required a good deal of sensitive questioning and ability to probe. The researcher developed these skills with the help of a pilot study which was carried out on eight families. This pilot study was used to refine the questionnaire and the researcher was encouraged to ask mothers to expand their answers. The researcher was responsible to a research team who were engaged in a number of different professional tasks but came together to guide the research, refine the methodology, analyse and discuss results. The research team comprised a child psychiatrist, a Bengali clinical psychologist, a social worker and a sociologist.

The researcher

A Sylheti-speaking research worker was employed to undertake the interviews. Since it was anticipated that the research would involve interviewing parents, mostly mothers in their homes, it was thought that a woman researcher would be more appropriate and acceptable to the Bangladeshis. The final choice from a shortlist of three compiled from an advertisement to which ten people responded was a university graduate in social psychology from the University of Dacca who had previously interviewed families in the area as part of an epidemiological study of risk factors for heart disease. Initially, the researcher, who did not live in Tower Hamlets, was apprehensive about travelling in the borough on her own because she feared racial attack. We arranged for her to be accompanied by a male medical student on her journeys and also gave her a personal alarm. This reassured her and she rapidly gained the confidence to travel on her own to families throughout the borough.

Selecting the sample

It was planned to interview more than 50 mothers and initially an attempt was made to contact them through community groups and women's groups which operated in Tower Hamlets. This proved quite difficult, since many groups fluctuated in size, especially in winter.

Finally, contact was achieved through children's clinics in some of the local GPs' surgeries. Once contacted, women were pleased to talk and gave the names of friends and acquaintances they thought would be willing to be interviewed. Of the 52 families contacted 49 were interviewed. The families were more likely to contain an employed husband (66 per cent) and most were social class 3, manual. Therefore, the group was atypical of the population, economically, since the employment rate was higher than the average for Bangladeshis in the borough (54 per cent).

We asked the interviewer to keep a diary of her reactions and experiences of interviewing. This diary proved useful in providing many practical points of detail about the accessibility of Bangladeshi women and the ease or difficulty of conducting interviews in small crowded dwellings where many children might be present. The interviews generally lasted over two hours and because of this two visits were usually needed.

Triangulation

The results of interviews were discussed by the research team at frequent intervals. When the interviews were completed and the material analysed, the findings were presented to a group of Muslim or Bangladeshi-speaking professionals, including social workers and a psychiatrist who worked in the borough. A further plan, to present the findings to a local Bangladeshi women's group has still to take place. The research team felt it important to triangulate the findings in this way.

The results: expectations of children

Table 3.1 Most frequently mentioned tasks expected of children at 4, 8 and 15 years of age

	Girls (%)	Boys (%)
4 years		
Carrying simple messages	44	40
Nothing	38	42
Tidying clothes	34	22
Looking at books	10	24
8 years		
Looking after siblings	82	74
Tidying clothes	72	54
Learning Arabic	68	64
Simple housework	62	62
Shopping	6	32
15 years		
Fasting	94	72
Cooking	78	8
Looking after siblings	46	76
Prayer	44	52
Studying carefully	30	42
Shopping	2	64

At early ages a substantial number of mothers did not have any particular expectations of children. Mainly, they mentioned tidiness or carrying a simple message: 'tell your father dinner is ready', 'call your brother'. Later, children became involved in looking after younger siblings and this responsibility continues, especially for boys, into adolescence. Boys have other particular duties, especially with regard to shopping. This reflects the greater male participation in shopping in this community. Only 2 per cent of women shop alone. The main household shopping is done by men. Boys are also expected to learn appropriate languages – Bengali and Arabic – and help parents in their relations with officials and others. There are higher domestic expectations for girls. They must have polite manners and entertain guests; however, boys are not excused domestic tasks. Children of both sexes are expected to be religious. Girls are not obliged to go to the mosque but they must fast. Boys are more likely to be involved in the external forms of religious worship – reciting the Qur'ān and attending the mosque (see Table 3.1).

These expectations of children have clear cultural and religious references but are similar to expectations of majority UK populations in that they imply a growing sense of development and responsibility. However, as one mother said:

Here you have to force children to have a religious education. Back home we did it automatically. Our children have to learn three things – English, Bengali, Arabic. English children only have to learn one thing.

Worrying behaviours

The sex differences observed in Table 3.2 show figures that reflect two rather different underlying features – on the one hand, some activities were mentioned as worrying because one sex is perceived

Table 3.2 Mothers' most frequently mentioned worrying behaviour in boys and girls

	Girls (%)	Boys (%)
4 years		
Soiling	64	50
Bed wetting	60	46
Overactive	40	44
Disobedience	30	30
Speech delay	18	8
Messy eating	20	4
Dangerous activities	6	14
8 years		
Disobedience	56	62
Truanting	42	32
Wanting to spend too much time outside	36	20
Careless about school work	20	32
Bed wetting	18	8
Fights with others	2	14
15 years		
Involvement with the opposite sex	36	36
Late home from school	24	36
Careless about school work	20	28
Truancy	14	20

as more likely to engage in them, e.g., boys and dangerous activities or fighting; on the other, because of a gendered view of worrying behaviour, it seems that issues of bodily control and development are more seriously regarded for younger girls. This was confirmed in discussions with Bengali-speaking professionals. Although the tables show most commonly mentioned forms of worrying behaviour many other aspects were also mentioned. For older boys in particular, the worries related to alcohol use, fighting (unsurprising considering the number of racist attacks in this part of London) and truancy. Mothers were concerned about the inability of girls to maintain the fasting rule, going out too much, being inconsiderate or unhelpful with housework and not observing purdah. Generally, parents were concerned about those aspects of children's, especially adolescents', behaviour which would bring them into conflict with the cultural expectations of their own group or with hostile members of the indigenous population:

> 'Children are not confined to the house so much in Bangladesh. There are open spaces for them to play. Here children are confined to rooms most of the time which helps to make them naughty.'

> 'I think I am verbally abused when I go out, which I sometimes understand, but I do not give replies. Sometimes because of my poor understanding I do not comprehend what they say.'

Help for worrying behaviours, naughtiness and deviant behaviour: social support

Only one-fifth of mothers had another female to help them in the household. One-third of women had visited another relative in the past month. The index of social support was limited because it did not include visits to the women, but it does suggest that social contact is more limited, because of location and fear of going out, than in Bangladesh. Low social support was correlated with the perception of more worrying behaviours in children ($p = 0.001$). Over half the women perceived support as limited and 8 per cent said they had no one to share problems with.

In cases of illness, doctors were the most favoured source of help, both in England and Bangladesh, followed by the mullah, although 12 per cent of mothers put the mullah first. Persons at the mosque, the hakim and the use of prayer were all considered important. In

Bangladesh, a traditional spiritual healer (pir) would also be consulted. Several mothers mentioned that both physical illnesses and what Western psychiatry regards as disordered behaviour in children may have a non-physical cause:

'There are certain illnesses that do not respond to medical treatments – for example, unexplained high temperature, fits, headaches – certain things like bed wetting at 14, or too much crying from a baby – these are caused by the influence of extra forces.'

'A mullah's treatment is needed when a child is possessed by certain influences. Their symptoms take the form of refusal of breast milk by a very young child, tendency of a child to alternate colour between black and white, being scared, screaming and crying.'

'If I feel it is a mullah's illness then I will go to the mullah. When we feel that doctors are unable to respond to a child's distress or illness, then we will go to the mullah.'

While the mullah was more likely to be consulted in Bangladesh, especially about emotional problems, his role is of considerable importance in England as well. There was a distinct suggestion that some matters were not amenable to medical ministration, although ultimately it was God who had the power to cure, whatever the intermediary. Nevertheless, even for these somewhat inexplicable occurrences, it seemed that in cases of unhappiness or disturbance, 48 per cent of mothers would contact a doctor, and 20 per cent the mullah. Sometimes mothers said they would go to both.

One mother made a very clear distinction between beliefs in Bangladesh and in England:

'I would just go to the doctor. No one else. You do not need a mullah or pir here. Are there mullahs and pirs here? I did not need them, because my children are not under the influence of anything "extra". I do not need water, talismans, a mullah for my children.'

But another said:

'I have a daughter of 10 who has a bed wetting problem. She wets at two- to three-day intervals. I have not spoken to the doctor about it – I have sought help from religious healers. I feel embarrassed to take her to the doctor on this issue.'

In common with the findings of other studies, these mothers saw parenting as an activity that established moral status. If children misbehaved or had other problems, this reflected on their parents. Although 'sickness' (however caused) was seen as at least partly the province of the doctor, children displaying 'naughtiness' and straightforward criminal behaviours like stealing would be taken first to relatives for advice and discipline. But even this step might be taken hesitantly. About one-fifth of mothers said they would try and deal with an emotional problem themselves:

'You cannot tell others. They will say "what can we do if you cannot control your own child?" I have seen underage children in this locality smoking, they do not care about their elders, youngsters drink and gamble and so forth.'

While in Bangladesh, mothers would consult with relations more readily, here they were less likely to do so or use only a limited number of relatives. Other sources of help mentioned were parents of children's friends or schoolteachers. From the mothers in our sample 20 per cent knew that there was a special profession that deals with children's worries, but most had not known that such a service existed. One mother remarked indignantly: 'My youngest child has terrible sleep problems, but our doctor does not refer him to these doctors.'

Comments

In terms of answering the original research question concerning underutilisation, the research offered some strong clues as to why so few children were referred to the clinic. As always with hindsight, more and better questions could have been asked.

A strong impression was conveyed via the interviews of a feeling of parental disempowerment in this society where legal statutes protecting children are highly developed compared to Bangladesh: 'They will say I am not adequate to look after a child, they might take away the child'. Services for children all carry a legal flavour and parents know this. At the same time, traditional sources of help in terms of female kin or a wider circle of relatives are not so readily available if problems with children emerge. Yet their British-born children were seen as potentially at risk:

'Birth place plays an important role in a person's life. You like the

things where you are born. A child born here does not like rice
and curry, he likes Western things.'

The dangers lay not only in threats to the accustomed way of life
but in the fears of racist attack and abuse. Although a highly spa-
tially integrated community is thought to provide security, this does
not necessarily relieve anxiety, merely extending the boundaries
of a haven.

Mothers seemed to convey a feeling of confusion and anxiety in
interviews about the society in which they were living. Their religious leaders and healers are a tried and tested means of assistance.
This needs to be more fully appreciated by professionals, who also
need to understand that the Western model of psychiatry which
they are using has important limitations, particularly in allowing a
universalism to its own observations that it denies to other systems.
That said, it was clear that many mothers simply were unaware of
the services that were available, and no effective means of publi-
cising them had been undertaken. In any case, their views about the
causes of children's bad or disturbed behaviour would not result in
choosing a psychiatric clinic for help. The same is true of white
families in Tower Hamlets. It is not suggested that the Bangladeshi
mothers strictly adhere to an alternative form of explanation of
behaviour and emotional difficulties but rather that a number of
explanations may be held at the same time on a temporary basis,
with notions about etiology being resolved retrospectively.

All mothers stressed the importance of sympathy and understanding to their children and themselves, and this had value whoever it came from. It is understandable that mothers might expect
these qualities to be more likely to be present in relatives and religious leaders or healers than in white, hospital-based professionals.
Conveying empathy is highly related to communication skills, which
in turn are assisted by a background of shared meanings and understandings. On these grounds, improving one's understanding of
another's culture or making professionally available those who do,
would seem to be an important part of providing a service for
children.

One example of good practice was as follows. A child from the
local Bangladeshi community was admitted to the hospital's acute
paediatric ward with a diagnosis of disturbed behaviour with acute
psychotic features. The child improved rapidly, responding to the
attention of a team of adults and to consistent handling of her

behaviour. The family brought in holy water from the mullah, read Qur'ānic verses over her bed and performed 'blows'. They were a deeply religious family and they attributed her improvement to their faith and observance of these rituals. However, they also acknowledged that the GP and child mental health team had made the right decision in facilitating admission, giving them a much-needed respite.

There does seem to be a need for the service that the Child and Family Consultation Service provides, as a 'third arm' which, together with the family and religious healers, helps to deal with the emotionally disturbed children of this community.

METHODOLOGICAL AND PRACTICAL ISSUES RAISED BY THE STUDY

The use of a questionnaire

The study was a combination of qualitative and quantitative approaches. A semi-structured questionnaire was used, with standard questions on age, number and sex of children, employment, social support and religious observance. Questions about childhood development and the perception of behavioural and emotional problems were open-ended, as were those on the perceptions of help and patterns of seeking help.

Two hypotheses linked the degree of social support and the degree of religious observance to the perception of worrying behaviours in children. Measurement of social support was limited and possibly invalid – simply the number of visits to relatives, perception of support for problems and help in the house. Nevertheless, some correlations were observed between a low level of social support and increased perception of worrying behaviour for 4- and 8-year-old boys ($p = 0.01$). The dependant variable 'worrying behaviours' was derived from each woman individually, from her own replies rather than ticking off a prepared list, and may have tapped differential amounts of knowledge or differential experience. In the whole sample the age range of children was wide, 60 per cent had one child in their family aged 11 to 15 or above, therefore most mothers would have had experience of the full developmental range of children.

The index of religious observance was produced by aggregating replies about religious practices (daily prayer, ritual cleanliness, fasting, etc.) and adherence to other observances – such as alms giving and pilgrimage. The index was probably a reasonable measure of devotion, but it was a mistake to use it as a proxy for 'traditional' values in the community. The possible relationship between traditional values and the likelihood or not of perceiving children's behaviours as problematic, remains theoretically confused. A better study of the salience of religious beliefs to health issues would need to explore this area more deeply. The index did not suggest a great deal of variation in the community in the degree of religious observance, in any case. However, what was learned from the index was that the religious dimension must not be overlooked in studying this community. For largely secular researchers, this involves a shift in mind-set.

Obtaining and conducting interviews

Generally speaking, the open-ended questions which sought qualitative data were quite successful and women spoke at length in response to them. It is impossible to know how far the fact that the interviewer was herself a Sylheti-speaking Muslim woman from Bangladesh contributed to the quality of information, but our guess is that these facts were fundamental to success. In her research notes, the interviewer listed a number of points which were essential to the good conduct of interviews, and to securing them in the first place.

- She was persistent. Most women lead busy lives with many commitments. Sometimes they were out when she arrived, or were asleep. Interview times had to be changed quite often, if a child was sick or an unexpected guest arrived. Yet most women were anxious to help and were always willing to try and rearrange times. She never gave up, and for this reason, the refusal rate in the study was very low.
- She was unhurried. She recognised the commitments of women, and always indicated that they should take their time. She noted that women were keen to be true to their word and insisted on giving interviews at the scheduled time, even when it brought difficulty on themselves.
- She sought rapport. She had a very gentle manner which put women at their ease. 'I found it useful to begin talking about the activities the families were engaged in . . . either a woman's involvement in cooking, a women's sense of satisfaction after buying a mirror or her worry about a child that was ill.'

- She was tactful. She always wore Muslim dress, but was careful
  that this should be simple and appropriate to the women she was
  visiting. Two problems she dealt with were negotiating the use of
  tape recorder and the presence of friends and relatives who also
  offered opinions. In the first instance, some women were embarrassed that they did not have mastery of standard Bengali and
  did not want to be recorded. The researcher assured them that
  she, as a Sylheti speaker, would be the only person listening to
  and transcribing the tapes, and that anonymity was guaranteed.
  In the second case, she politely noted responses, although emphasising that she was mainly interviewing a particular woman.
  During one interview she relates an incident where she was
  confronted: 'Halfway through interviewing one woman, her em-
  ployer, who supplies her with machine work and also claimed to
  be a community leader arrived. He advised me not to interview
  these women, "who do not know and are unaware about what is
  happening in their life", and not to use the tape recorder. He
  expressed cynicism about the so-called researchers whom he feels
  have been used to enhance the stereotypes about this vulnerable
  community. He also expresssed his concern about anyone doing
  anything in Tower Hamlets. By this he meant people claiming to
  be Sylheti or working as interpreters for Sylheti people, people
  without research training who are doing research. At last he
  agreed that I could continue interviewing the woman but said I
  should not use the tape recorder. He advised me to interview only
  those women who are aware about the issues that concern their
  life.' The researcher noted that she did not wish to offend the
  man, since she did not want to harm the employment chances of
  the woman she was interviewing. However, she suggested that if
  the man felt so strongly he should contact the psychiatrist or
  sociologist member of the research team who would be happy to
  come and discuss the research with him. So far he has not
  contacted them.
- She gave information and support. Many families said they were
  experiencing problems with their children and wanted advice
  from her. She listened to them and talked with them, and also
  gave them a leaflet printed in Bengali about the Child and Family
  Consultation Service. The leaflet encourages parents to phone
  directly if they are worried about their children. Many people
  had general complaints about the NHS, which it was agreed
  should be included in the final report.

CONCLUSIONS

This research has demonstrated that the concerns of individuals can be more readily understood when placed in their cultural context. This does not deny the impact of material factors and hostile environmental conditions on their lives. It does, however, enable us to see how these pressures are articulated and understood. Above all, it suggests the complexity of the experience of migrant groups and draws attention to the lack of sensitive research in this area.

In the beginning we sought an answer to an apparently simply question. In so doing, we uncovered numerous others. What are the main forces for socialising children into a society different to that in which their parents were born? What is the nature of parental influence? Is there a crisis over the management of children, or is this just an example of 'moral panic'? Is the concept of 'community' useful in this research or does it impose unrealistic homogeneity to a group fractured by unemployment? How clear and extensive are culturally distinct health beliefs? Do they change, and if so where and when? How can services be publicised? How can they be made culturally appropriate? We learnt nothing that suggested the existence of psychiatric pathology on a large scale that was going unidentified; such information would need a different kind of study in any case. What resulted was a series of pointers on which a better service could be built.

If the purpose of research is to generate new questions rather than to answer old ones, then this has been achieved. Certainly, in health care delivery the problems that need to be solved are unlikely to be so narrowly focused as the original research question. The combination of both qualitative and quantitative methodologies and the attempt to monitor and discuss results with Muslim professionals has been a way to test the 'resonance' of our findings. Such an approach was necessary in order to identify whether or not cultural differences in health beliefs and expectations existed, and if they did, how relevant these differences might be. The challenge now is to translate those findings into appropriate clinical practice.

ACKNOWLEDGEMENTS

Dr Ruma Bhose (Child and Family Consultation Service), Afreem Huq, Rosemary Loshak and Dr Frances Marks (Child and Family

Consultation Service). Ferdouzi Choudhry, Ruma Sabe (NSPCC), Kesseoa Opoku, Afreen Rashid Islam, Sukuti Sen, Farida Hassan and Nadina Osmany (Stepney Social Services).

REFERENCES

Abdullah, T. A. and Zeidenstein, S. A. (1982) *Village Women of Bangladesh: Prospects for Change*. Oxford: Pergamon Press.

Adams, C. (1994) *Across Seven Seas and Thirteen Rivers*. London: Eastside Books.

Ahmad, W. (1993) *'Race' and Health in Contemporary Britain*. Buckingham: Open University Press.

Bagley, C. (1971) 'The social etiology of schizophrenia in immigrant groups', *International Journal of Social Psychiatry* 17: 292–304.

Bal, S. (1986) 'The symptomatology of mental illness among Asians in the West Midlands' (BA dissertation, Wolverhampton Polytechnic), quoted in A. Hopkins and V. Bhal (1993) *Access to Health Care for People from Black and Ethnic Minorities*. London: Royal College of Physicians.

Balarajan, R. and Raleigh, V. S. (1993) *Ethnicity and Health: a Guide for the NHS*. London: Department of Health.

Banatvala, N. and Jayaratnam, J. (1995) 'The experience of East London's minority ethnic community', *Health in the East End: Annual Public Health Report 1995/1996*. London: Department of Public Health, East London and City Health Authority.

Beliappa J. (1991) *Illness or Distress? Alternative Models of Mental Health*. London: Confederation of Indian Organisations (UK).

Bhana, K. (1986) 'Indian indigenous healers', *South African Medical Journal* 70 (4): 221–223.

Bhatt, T. A., Thomenson, B. and Benjamin, S. (1989) 'Transcultural patterns of somatisation in primary care', *Journal of Psychosomatic Research* 33: 671–680.

Bhattacharya, D. P. (1986) *Paglami: Ethnopsychiatric Knowledge in Bengal* (Foreign and Comparative East Asian Studies No. 11). Syracuse, NY: Syracuse University, Maxwell School of Citizenship in Public Affairs.

Bridges, K. W., Goldberg, N. P. (1985) 'Somatic presentation of DSM III psychiatric disorders in primary care', *Journal of Psychosomatic Research* 29: 563–569.

Centre for Bangladeshi Studies (1994) *Routes and Beyond*. London: Centre for Bangladeshi Studies.

Cochrane, R. and Bal, S. (1989) 'Mental hospital admission rates of immigrants to England: a comparison of 1971 and 1981', *Social Psychiatry and Epidemiology* 24: 2–11.

Cochrane, R. and Stopes Roe, M. (1977) 'Psychological and social adjustment of Asian immigrants to Britain', *Social Psychiatry* 12: 195–207.

Currer, C. and Stacey, M. (eds) (1991) *Concepts of Health, Illness and Disease*. Oxford: Berg.

ELCHA (East London and City Health Authority) (1995) *Health in the East End*. London: Department of Public Health Medicine/ELCHA.

Fernando, S. (1991) *Mental Health, Race and Culture*. Basingstoke: Macmillan.

Francis, E. (1993) 'Psychiatric racism and social police: black people and the psychiatric services' in W. James and C. Harris (eds) *Inside Babylon: the Caribbean Diaspora in Britain*. London: Verso.

Hackett, L. Hackett, R. and Taylor, D. C. (1991) 'Psychological disturbance and its associations in the children of the Gujarati community', *Journal of Clinical Psychology and Psychiatry* 32: 851–856.

Hillier, S., Loshak, R., Marks, F. and Rahman, S. (1994) 'An evaluation of child psychiatric services for Bangladeshi parents', *Journal of Mental Health* 3: 327–337.

Howlett, B., Ahmad, W. and Murray, R. (1992) 'An explanation of White, Asian and Afro-Caribbean people's concepts of health and illness causation', *New Community* 18(2): 281–292.

Kallarackal, A. M. and Herbert, M. (1976) 'The happiness of Indian immigrant children', *New Society* 4: 22–24.

Kleinman, A. (1987) 'Culture and clinical reality: commentary on culture-bound syndromes and international disease classifications', *Culture, Medicine and Psychiatry* 11: 49–52.

Littlewood, R. (1992) 'Psychiatric diagnosis and racial bias: empirical and interpretative approaches', *Social Science and Medicine* 34(2): 141–149.

Littlewood, R. and Lipsedge, M. (1989) *Aliens and Alienists*. London: Unwin Hyman.

Loring, M. and Powell, B. (1988) 'Gender race and DSM III: A study of the objectivity of psychiatric diagnostic behaviours', *Journal of Health and Social Behaviour* 29: 1–22.

McCormick, A. and Rosenbaum, M. (1990) *1981–1992 Morbidity Statistics from General Practice* (Third National Study Socio-economic analysis Series M85 2). London: HMSO.

Marks, F. M. (1994) 'A survey of psychological problems of ethnic minority and indigenous children in Tower Hamlets Schools' (unpublished), Child and Family Consultation Service/Royal Hospitals NHS Trust.

Marmot, M., Adelstein, A. and Bulusu, L. (1984) 'Immigrant mortality in England and Wales 1970–78' in *Studies in Medical and Population Subjects* 47, London: HMSO.

Newth, S. J. and Corbett, J. (1993) 'Behaviour and emotional problems in three year old children of Asian parentage', *Journal Child Psychology and Psychiatry* 34: 333–352.

Nichter, M. (1981) 'Negotiation of the illness experience: Ayurvedic therapy and the psychosocial dimension of illness', *Culture Medicine and Psychiatry* 5: 5–24.

Parmar, P. (1981) 'Young Asian women: a critique of the pathological approaches', *Multiracial Education* 3: 19–25.

Pearson, M. (1983) *Ethnic Minority Studies: Friend or Foe?* Bradford: Centre for Ethnic Minority Health Studies.

Phizacklea, A. and Miles, R. (1979) 'Working-class racist beliefs in the inner city' in R. Miles and A. Phizacklea (eds) *Racism and Political Action in Britain*. London: Routledge and Kegan Paul.

Pilgrim, D. and Rogers, A. (1993) *A Sociology of Mental Health and Illness*. Buckingham: Open University Press.

Rutter, M. and Giller, H. (1983) *Juvenile Deliquency: Trends and Perspectives*. Harmondsworth: Penguin.

Silman, A., Loysen, E., De Graaf, W. and Sramek, M. (1985) 'High dietary fat intake and cigarette smoking as risk factors for ischaemic heart disease in Bangladeshi male immigrants in East London', *Journal of Epidemiology and Community Health* 39 (41): 152–155.

Smaje, C. (1995) *Health Race and Ethnicity: Make Sense of the Evidence*. London: King's Fund Institute.

Srinivasa, D. K. and Trivedi, S. (1982) 'Knowledge of and attitudes to mental diseases in a rural community in South India', *Social Science and Medicine* 16: 1635–1639.

Stern, G., Cottrell, D. and Holmes, J. (1990) 'Patterns of attendance of child psychiatry out patients with special reference to Asian families', *British Journal of Psychiatry* 156: 384–387.

Tower Hamlets Education (1991) *Pupil Language Census 1991–2*. London: Education Strategy Group.

Tunstall-Pedoe, H., Claydon, D., Morris, J., Brigden, W. and McDonald, L. (1975) 'Coronary heart disease attacks in East London', *Lancet* 2: 833–836.

Vanstraelan, M., Marks, F. and Hillier, S. (1996) 'A comparative evaluation of British indigenous and British Bangladeshi families referred to a child psychiatry service in East London' (in press).

Chapter 4

A defence of the use of the terms 'ethnicity' and 'culture'

David Kelleher

INTRODUCTION

There is a debate about how we should characterise the differences between groups in contemporary societies such as England. It is clear to the eye of any observer on the street, in hospitals or in people's homes that there are many differences between people in present-day England, but what differences should we pay attention to and how should we characterise those differences? As with all observation, what we see depends on the theoretical framework or sensitising notions we start with. But that is not to say that what we see depends purely on a technical decision about which theoretical concepts we decide to use to see with; there are also political considerations which influence the choice of concepts and the meanings we ascribe to them. For analytical purposes it is important to clarify what political perspectives attach to the words 'race' and 'class' on the one hand and culture and ethnicity on the other, but this is also important for practical purposes in relation to how we explain the links between these concepts and health. This chapter will argue that there is both theoretical validity and practical usefulness in using the concepts of culture and ethnicity in understanding differences in health. One broad way in which we can characterise the debate about how we should view the differences we can see is to say that the debate is between those who argue that there are broad similarities which are shared by all those people who are non-white and those who argue that there may be significant differences between the many ethnic groups within the whole range of non-white and white groups. Those who put forward the former view claim that because of the racism that non-white people experience, the position of all black people in terms of their economic position, life chances and health is likely to be similar, and also poorer than the economic position, life chances and health of white people living in England (Kushnick 1988). Those who say that they see diversity and a range of ethnic groups do not deny that many of these ethnic groups experience racism and have the similar experiences of structural pressures, which affect their life chances, economic position and health, but they suggest that the culture of these groups may also be important in influencing how they respond to and manage their situation. They would also argue that ethnic groups are not necessarily defined by their colour. The attempt to equate ethnic minority status with being 'black' seems to stem from a crude Marxist position and a form of classification which glosses over many differences between groups in order to achieve a political unity around what is seen as a 'real' similarity of economic interest, as opposed to a concern with superficial differences of culture (Modood 1994). The view taken here will be similar to that expressed by Rex (1986) who describes his position as being Weberian. He argues that:

> Class theory can and should be supplemented by the theory of ethnicity. At the same time, the theory of ethnicity should recognise that collective ethnic organization may lie dormant and only become activated by the emergence of shared interests.
>
> (Rex 1986: 81)

The debate which will be described in this chapter is therefore about the relative importance to be attached to ethnicity and culture in understanding the health and illness of people from what can be called ethnic minority groups. There will also be some discussion of the value of and problems associated with carrying out ethnographic research among ethnic minority groups, for as Smaje (1995) points out, one important issue is how research is carried out, as well as how relevant it is for health policy decision-making.

Before examining in more detail the arguments about the use of the terms 'culture' and 'ethnicity', it is necessary to make some preliminary clarification of how they will be used, and how the position taken here relates to the work of other writers in this area. The view here is that these terms have been used in differing ways and given greater importance at some times than others. The consequence is that ethnic differences, unlike racial differences, are not viewed as being essentialist; they are, as Barth (1969) and Wallman

(1986) have argued, constructed differences which have as much to do with groups constructing boundaries between themselves and others as they have with their being labelled as 'Other' by dominant groups. Brah, in a review article (1994), notes how the meaning of 'the term "ethnic" has varied from being a polite way of referring to Jews, Italians, Irish and other groups in contrast to the dominant group [in the USA] of largely English descent' (Brah, 1994: 810) to the situation in post-war England, where the term has been mainly used by white English to describe non-white people from Africa, the Asian subcontinent and the Caribbean and their English-born children. European minority groups living in England have had to claim ethnic status in order to obtain political and economic benefits offered by the state.

While ethnicity has therefore been a way of describing groups seen as inferior, it has also been used by other groups to claim that their relationship to the dominant group has been a common experience of oppression/subordination. This experience has encouraged such groups as the Irish to argue that they also have a culture which is distinct from that of the English and that they constitute an ethnic minority.

'Culture' is a less problematic term, although it can be defined minimally as a set of beliefs and ideas that a group draws on to identify and manage the problems of their everyday lives or, more extensively, to include history, laws, artefacts, art and literature as well. The important point to emphasise in relation to understanding how people perceive health and illness is to recognise that culture is a dynamic entity which changes to incorporate fresh ideas and perspectives as people develop new ways of responding to their environment.

ARGUMENTS AGAINST ETHNICITY AND CULTURAL ANALYSIS

The arguments of those who oppose the use of the categories of culture and ethnicity, and the exploration of difference, often described as anti-racists (Smaje 1995), are put forward by Waqar Ahmad in Chapter 9 of this volume, so it is only necessary to summarise some of them here. A number of writers (Pearson 1983; Donovan 1986; Ahmad 1993) make the argument that cultural analysis is a diversion from the more important issue of showing how racism is a common experience of all black (non-white) people and that this is the major factor involving them in social disadvantage and often a higher rate of illness from a range of diseases. Ahmad states the argument very clearly:

> A major issue in the racialization of health research is that it is assumed that the populations can be meaningfully divided into 'ethnic' or 'racial' groups, taking these as primary categories and using these categories for explanatory purposes. Stratification by class, income and so on is then seen as unimportant; issues of institutional and individual racism as determinants of health status or healthcare become peripheral at best.
>
> (Ahmad 1993: 19)

It is also suggested that cultural analysis emphasises the distinguishing features of ethnic minority groups, ignoring their common experience and the differences within any one ethnic group. Brah, for example suggests that:

> Ethnicism, I would suggest, defines the experience of racialised groups primarily in 'culturalist' terms: that is, it posits 'ethnic difference' as the primary modality around which social life is constituted and experienced. Cultural needs are defined largely as independent of other social experiences centred around class, gender, racism or sexuality. This means that a group identified as culturally different is assumed to be internally homogenous.
>
> (Brah 1992: 129)

Anti-racists also argue that culturally based research using ethnicity as the independent variable has not led to much improvement of services for black people or to an improvement in their health status (Pearson 1983; Ahmad 1993). This view may be attributable to the structuralist position they propose, in which, to varying degrees, they ignore the small-scale developments and improvements in attitudes that have taken place. Awareness of cultural practices has allowed health workers to develop a campaign related to the period of fasting for Ramadan to encourage people to give up smoking after Ramadan as well as for that month (Directorate of Public Health, ELCHA 1995/6). This is an important initiative as there is a high rate of smoking and chewing tobacco amongst some Muslim groups. In addition to such small-scale projects which are based on knowledge of cultural differences, it is interesting to note the sensitivity to cultural differences and to the complexities of ethnicity shown in the British Medical Association publication,

Multicultural Health Care (1995). As well as recognising the need for epidemiological research, it supports the need for more research which would improve doctors' awareness of the different approaches to health, illness and death within various cultures. The publication also accepts that ethnicity is not something which is fixed but something which may change according to context and that economic and social deprivation are important factors affecting health.

Smaje (1995) has produced an excellent summary of a range of recent research findings which forms a useful contribution to understanding the importance of both cultural and material factors. He has also drawn attention to the difficulties involved in distinguishing material and cultural factors in health and the problem of defining ethnic groupings. He suggests that whilst it cannot be said that the evidence produced by culturally sensitive research has clearly shown the validity of this approach for policy-making, more such research is needed. Such research should attempt to produce 'more refined approaches to the dynamic interactions between culture, socioeconomic status and health experience' (Smaje 1995: 124–125). He makes a similar point in discussing the usefulness of materialist explanations, and reports that evidence from the more extensive US literature is inconclusive about whether socio-economic status alone can account for 'racial' disparities in health.

CONCEPTUAL PROBLEMS IN USING THE TERMS 'ETHNICITY' AND 'CULTURE'

The argument cannot easily be settled by more research, however; there are clearly conceptual and political differences which will continue to guide both the practices of researchers, the interpretation of their findings, and the ways in which these findings are used. Being aware of the criticisms made by anti-racists of culturally based research can at least make such researchers alert to the need to place their study of a particular ethnic group within a wider context. In time, anti-racist researchers may also come to appreciate that ethnic differences can be used positively in ways that take account of how people in ethnic minority groups see themselves. Before such a *rapprochement* can take place, the process of clarifying the differences between the positions needs to continue. Anti-racist writers, for example, claim that research focusing on the culture of a particular ethnic group tends to show the negative aspects of that culture in relation to health or to describe exotic elements in it (Donovan 1986). This approach is also part of a process of constructing the people in ethnic minority groups as 'Other' (Ahmad 1993), pointing to elements of a lifestyle which differ from what is assumed to be a 'normal' English lifestyle (Pearson 1983; Donovan 1986). Sashidharan and Francis (1993), in discussing the epidemiological data which indicates a link between ethnicity and schizophrenia, suggest that the self of the European is strengthened by the implicit linking of madness with the 'Other', the different and irrational non-European black person. Senior and Bhopal (1994) show how such ethnocentrism can be detected in what is apparently straightforward epidemiological work. They give as an example earlier findings about mortality rates in men from the Indian subcontinent. When standardised mortality rates are used, which compare an ethnic minority group with the general population, it can be shown that the ethnic minority group has a high rate for certain diseases. Senior and Bhopal argue that if the number of deaths is compared, then a different picture appears; what may be seen then is that most deaths in males from the Indian subcontinent are caused by heart disease and this is, in fact, similar to the general population, not different from it. They argue that it is important to identify the major causes of death in ethnic minority populations rather than looking for causes of death which are high in the minority group in comparison with the general population. Such research points to differences which may be real but are, in policy terms, less significant than the similarities.

It can be argued that the process of describing difference is not simply one of distinguishing between groups in a neutral way, but is implicitly making a point about inferiority and superiority. Such description of differences then becomes a new form of racism. Goldberg (1993) states the position in this way:

> the cultural conception of race has tended to eclipse all other. It has become paradigmatic. But it has also largely suppressed heirarchical judgements of inferiority and superiority as the basis of exclusions, coding the exclusions it promotes in terms merely of racial difference. This raises a fundamental question about the cultural conception. Many insist that racial differentiation inevitably appeals, if only implicitly, to underlying biological claims . . . Thus the only difference, if any, between 19th century and 20th

century forms of racial differentiation seems on this reading to
be at the level of surface expression.

(Goldberg 1993: 71)

Goldberg goes on to argue that 'ethnic reduction' first constructs
all ethnic minorities as similar; they represent the 'Other', but the
'Other' is then disaggregated as some are seen as making progress
towards assimilation while others are blamed for failing to do so.
The groups that are seen as failing to do so fail, it is suggested,
because of the values of their culture rather than as a result of their
history and experience. In this way the culture of the group is
pathologised.

This argument, that the description of ethnic minority cultures is
implicitly ethnocentric and that within the tradition of European
anthropology there has been, as Fanon (1986) argues, a way of
seeing the differences as differences from the normal, civilised European culture, is an argument which has to be taken seriously. It is
not one which cannot be overcome however, for although Goldberg
(1993) suggests that the process of naming the 'Other' and therefore
the naming of ethnic groups is something which is done to these
groups, as is the case in epidemiological research, there is the
counter-argument which stresses the role that groups play in
naming themselves. This can be shown in ethnographic research
such as that conducted by Modood, Beishon and Virdee (1994)

Another objection, practical this time rather than political, that is
raised in relation to the use of ethnic groupings is the problem of
defining the boundaries of ethnic groups and deciding who is and
who is not a member of a particular group. McKenzie and Crowcroft
(1994), in arguing against using ethnicity as a variable in health
research, show the crudity of many of the ethnic classifications
which are in use. The ethnicity classification is most problematic in
relation to second- and third-generation people whose parents came
to Britain as immigrants but who themselves may have been born in
England and been educated here, and have English accents. They
may also have had considerable contact with an English culture.
There are grounds for including such people as members of their
parents' ethnic group, as Raftery, Jones and Rosato (1990) show in
relation to the Irish (see Chapter 6 in this volume). It may be that
membership of that group, although a part of their experience, is
less central to their identity because they may have moved out of
the community into which they were born as a result of education

and socio-economic change. In that case they may have come to regard their occupation as more significant in terms of their identity but still cling to what Nagel (1994) describes as 'symbolic ethnicity'. Hall (1992a) in fact goes further and suggests that the postmodern subject has no fixed identity: 'The fully unified, completed, secure and coherent identity is a fantasy' (Hall 1992a: 277). Although we may construct a narrative of the self to comfort ourselves, the reality is that we often have contradictory identities within us which we use in different situations. It may be, therefore, that ethnicity is only one strand in the identity of second-generation people, but this will also be discussed later.

The case of second-generation people is just one example of the difficulties there can be in deciding the boundaries of an ethnic group. There is also the question of the appropriateness of categories such as 'Asian'. First, categories such as 'Asian' are not describing a homogenous group and such a categorisation may mean something different in different places (in the USA, for example, it is likely to refer to the Japanese) or at different times. It is also important to note that, as Nagel (1994) says:

> The location and meaning of particular ethnic boundaries are continuously negotiated, revised and revitalized, both by ethnic group members as well as by outside observers.
>
> (Nagel 1994: 153)

For a number of reasons it is the case that the ethnic labels used by others may be crude or even inaccurate indications of what the people so labelled share, what their ethnicity means to them. It is important to explore this and to deconstruct the certainty which is implicit in categories used in most epidemiological research.

ETHNICITY AND CULTURE IN THE CONSTRUCTION OF IDENTITY

If we accept a nominalist position, the differences between the people in different ethnic groups are not of an essentialist kind; unlike 'racial' differences, which those who use such categories believe reflect underlying genetic traits. The argument now becomes one that says that ethnic differences are constructed differences. In the past, ethnic identities may have reflected colonialism's preoccupation with the 'Other'. Today in the USA and England, dominant groups still play an important part in the production of ethnic labels. Yet at the same time, individuals and the groups they identify with play a part in the ongoing process of constructing ethnicity and ethnic identities. And although ethnic groupings have been described as 'imagined communities' (Anderson 1983) and members of them may be torn by the sometimes contradictory identities they hold (Hall 1992a), they do have very real and practical uses for people as well. Max Weber noted both of these points when he stated that:

> The belief in group affinity, regardless of whether it has any objective foundation, can have important consequences especially for the formation of a political community. We shall call 'ethnic groups' those human groups that entertain a subjective belief in their common descent because of similarities of physical type or of customs or both, or because of memories of colonization and migration
>
> (Weber 1968: 389)

Whilst it is accepted, therefore, that differences in class are major determinants of how people live, and that ethnic and cultural differences may be less important than class or socio-economic position in explaining differences in health status, the argument here is (following Rex 1986) that ethnicity and culture are still important. They are important because to some extent they are self-maintained structures which have significance for both individuals and the political ambitions of the group. Although Donovan states that 'On the whole, individuals have been considered to be subsumed within their cultures and have been afforded little autonomy' (Donovan 1986: 42), the view taken here is not to regard people in ethnic minority groups as 'cultural dopes' (Garfinkel 1984: 68) who live unproblematically by simply following the taken-for-granted rules of their culture, but as people actively playing a part in the construction of their ethnicity by trying to reconcile and integrate the sometimes conflicting structures of relevance (Schutz 1966) in their lives. This is a symbolic interactionist perspective and is the view taken by Nagel (1994) who stresses the point that culture and ethnicity often become the focus of political negotiation and struggle for groups as well as ethnic identity being an organising concept for individuals trying to find where they fit into a changing and often hostile world. Some of the empirical studies in this book illustrate the similarity in the experiences of 'different' ethnic groups, but others draw attention to the importance of their culture and ethnicity for the people in those groups. It is not just that dominant groups construct people into ethnic groups; people do this for themselves.

In addition, they may also see themselves as members of a wider, more inclusive grouping than an ethnic group, and this may be one of the other structures of relevance that they struggle with. It may be, as some anti-racists argue, that many members of ethnic minority groups see themselves as 'black', and being black becomes something which they choose to make an organising notion for their political activity and an important structure of relevance for themselves in making sense of the experience of their ongoing lives, including their experience of health services. Their typifications of other people and their definitions of situations may be based on seeing people as black and like themselves or white and therefore different. However, it should not be assumed that people do see themselves as black, for, as Brah (1992) notes, although the concept may have political significance for South Asian people, it denies them their cultural identity; many of them would see being Muslim as being a more important structure of relevance shaping both how others see them and how they define themselves. Modood, Beishon and Virdee (1994) report that in their study, and in others, being Muslim was at the core of their identity for people from Pakistan and Bangladesh. It is likely that the typifications of many, but not all, people who are Muslim, start from seeing themselves as Muslim people and others as not, rather than seeing themselves as black and others not, or themselves as Bengali and others not. In other words, their identity may be not be built around a sense of nationality nor on the experience of being non-white, but from seeing themselves as members of Islam, an attachment which crosses national boundaries and ethnic ones.

It is important to recognise that while the argument here is that ethnic identity is something which is constructed by people themselves, they do not have a free hand in this; external influences may construct people as black in spite of their desire to see themselves as English or Indian or Muslim. Goldberg (1993) expresses the view that we do have some choice in terms of our national identity, although that choice may well be constrained by race, class and circumstance. Nagel (1994) gives more emphasis to the constructionist view while still recognising that there are external and political constraints:

Ethnic identity, then, is the result of a dialectical process involving internal and external opinions and processes, as well as the individual's self-identification and outsiders' ethnic designations.

(Nagel 1994: 154)

Modood (1994) suggests that while earlier immigrants, such as the Jews and the Irish, have tended to play down their ethnic backgrounds in public and have been able to do this relatively successfully, but at some cost to themselves, people from non-European ethnic backgrounds have been less able to escape the external, public influence on their identity. Racists in society are inclined to lump together all non-white people as 'black', and it has sometimes seemed as though immigration policies also discriminate in this way, when distinctions are drawn between 'old' Commonwealth countries and 'new' Commonwealth countries, for example. Being a Muslim also has a more public aspect to it than being a Catholic or Jew. For many Muslims it entails wearing a particular form of dress. This may be the case for some Jews, but it is not so for the majority.

Not only are people with a non-white ethnic background likely to have less choice in terms of their identity because they are not able to avoid the public, external constraints in the construction of it, as their skin colour marks them out as different, but many of them do not choose to hide their ethnic identity. Although in the 1970s assimilation was the aim of public policy, many groups resisted this and sought to retain their culture and ethnic identity. This led to the development of a policy of multiculturalism.

One reason why people may choose to stress an ethnic element in their identity and see being a member of an ethnic group as important is that by so doing they gain a sense of community. Bauman (1992) describes the contemporary world as a postmodern place where fears are privatised. A common response is for people to retreat into 'tribalism', a move which he sees as understandable but perilous if difference is not seen as 'the equivalence of knowledge-producing discourses' (Bauman 1992: xxi).

The contemporary situations in Northern Ireland and in the former Yugoslavia, where people build their identities and sense of community around ethnicity and draw the boundaries very fiercely around themselves, excluding others, show both the reality and the dangers of tribalism.

At an empirical and individual level Modood, Beishon and Virdee (1994) illustrate another less threatening aspect of what

Bauman may mean by a retreat into tribalism when they also describe the benefits that older people from a Caribbean background felt when they were in community groups made up of people like themselves rather than in multi-ethnic groups. They felt, like the people in the carers' groups for Bengali and Chinese in the East End of London, 'more at home'. And the feeling that they are one of a group may give them a sense of security when faced with the changing contingencies in what is often an alien and sometimes violently hostile world. That is not to say that it is always simply a case of people rediscovering a historically constructed culture and ethnicity, for, as commentators as different as Rattansi (1992) and Bhabba (1994) have pointed out, the culture that they embrace may well include in it new elements adapted from the 'host' society. To return to the main argument of this chapter, though, it is the case that, as Bhabba puts it:

> The great connective narratives of capitalism and class drive the engines of social reproduction, but do not, in themselves provide a foundational frame for those modes of cultural identification and political affect that form around issues of sexuality, race, feminism, the lifeworld of refugees or migrants.
>
> (Bhabba 1994: 6)

Hall, in an article called 'New ethnicities' (1992b), also argues that while politically it has been important for non-white people from ethnic minorities to see themselves as 'black', there is now a case for recognising diversity and difference, and the concept which allows this is 'ethnicity':

> If the black subject and black experience are not stabilized by Nature or by some other essential guarantee, then it must be the case that they are constructed historically, culturally, politically – and the concept which refers to this is 'ethnicity'.
>
> (Hall 1992b: 226)

There is, then, a recognised need that immigrant people and their children may have, a need to identify with others who are seen as being like themselves in some way and to find in the culture they share and create a sense of community. Whether it is a real community in the sense that it is for the Bangladeshi people living in the East End of London, who live close together, setting up the shops and mosques which help to sustain their way of life, or whether it is an 'imagined' community which has a symbolic meaning, in the sense that it is used by Bauman (1992), it may be a source of strength and comfort to people who feel they are regarded by others as different. Being regarded as different may lead to people becoming more aware of their ethnicity and cultural identity. Recognising their difference and turning it into a source of strength is one reason why people may emphasise cultural differences in terms of what they eat and how they dress, and this may lead them to maintaining an allegiance to the religion of their group and to become even more aware of what it is to be a Muslim than are the people in Bangladesh. This is one of the paths which some young, second-generation Bangladeshi people are taking. So, while for some their religion has become the most important structure of relevance in their lives, for others a more important focus for their life may be being a student, or a businessman or a doctor. The book *Routes and Beyond*, subtitled 'Voices from educationally successful Bangladeshis', illustrates well the range of identity issues which concern young Bangladeshis. One says: 'In two years time there is a council election coming up and that's one target' (Centre for Bangladeshi Studies 1994: 41). Another says:

I think every Muslim woman and man who can afford to and who are mature and believe that they can take the responsibility of getting married, should get married
(Centre for Bangladeshi Studies, 1994: 43)

Ethnicity and culture may become part of a resistance to the experience of racism or discrimination. This point is accepted by those who might broadly be said to be anti-racist rather than multiculturalist. Donovan (1986) for example, refers to the case of Hasidism among Jews and of Rastafarianism among Afro-Caribbean people. Modood, Beishon and Virdee (1994) make the point that:

In conditions of insecurity it is not surprising if individuals and communities cling to and assert what gives them psychological strength. These forms of insecure assertiveness can raise the political profile of the minority or minorities in question. But it can itself lead to increased majority hostility and stimulate more rejectionism.
(Modood, Beishon and Virdee 1994: 105)

They go on to warn that attempts to identify oneself with the majority group may also lead to rejection.

Another reason why people define themselves as an ethnic group is that it provides them with a way of making a claim for resources (Modood, Beishon and Virdee 1994). While some (see, for example, Ahmad and Sheldon 1992) argue that it is not helpful to collect ethnic statistics, it can be argued that many people from ethnic minority backgrounds do experience difficulty in obtaining adequate housing and fare badly in terms of employment and in the treatment that they receive from the social security and health care systems relative to their need. The collection of such statistics highlights these inequalities. These problems affect the lives of the second and third generations as well as those who came as immigrants. One reason why the Irish in England have sought recognition as an ethnic minority is to overcome their statistical invisibility (Bhrolchain 1990) and the cultural insensitivity they experience in health and social sevices (Bagley and Binitie 1970; Perkins 1994). Nagel (1994) describes how groups in the USA have shaped their ethnic identities to take advantage of affirmative action programmes. She also gives as an example the case of the 'Untouchables' in India, arguing that a similar process led to 'Untouchables' from different language and regional backgrounds developing a collective identity. This could be seen as a caste-based movement rather than an ethnic grouping. A clear example of a group which has emphasised its ethnic differences and culture in order to claim a distinctive niche and a better share of resources is the case of Scots in Britain who have formed the Scottish National Party. They have emphasised their difference and put the question of devolution for Scotland firmly on the political agenda in order to try to gain what they see as a fairer share of resources for Scottish people.

Researchers who want to use the concepts of culture and ethnicity do not believe, however, that in constructing an ethnicity and culture people are simply taking over a fully formed monolithic set of rules for living; it is rather that the 'inherited' culture is what they see people as sharing and this is what forges them into a group to face the common problems they experience. But the process of culturally based research is not one of digging up a past culture in order to be able to predict precisely in a positivist way what people believe and how they will behave; it is guided by an awareness of some of the problems people in particular ethnic minority groups currently face and a desire to know more about how they perceive their situation and how they are using their cultural resources to address their current problems. On a practical level it is necessary for health care workers to know for example the broad outlines of the kind of foods eaten by a particular cultural group in order to be able to ask individuals about their diet. It is also useful to know whether the reasons why people consume or avoid particular foods are cultural or religious. It may be easier to talk to people about making adjustments to their diet, such as changing from white bread to brown bread, if you know that the reason why they buy white bread is because they believe that a certain brand of white bread is free from animal fats and is therefore halal.

Such knowledge of the ongoing and developing culture of ethnic minority groups can be seen as useful in that it provides us all with information about the diversity of values, beliefs and practices within ethnic groups, as well as between them, in contemporary society. The attitudes, beliefs and behaviour of people in the wider society, including health care professionals tend to be based on limited experience and the stereotypical views of ethnic minority people conveyed in the mass media. Bowler (1993) in her study of how midwives used stereotypes in their perceptions of mothers of South-Asian descent shows how this may work. She suggests that the stereotypes used by the midwives led to the 'Asian' mothers in the study being disadvantaged in the treatment and care they received. Bowler goes on to suggest that 'cultural awareness training' may contribute to the production of stereotypes, but I would argue that this should not be so if the cultural awareness itself avoids stereotyping and shows the complexity of identity formation as suggested in this chapter.

Therefore, the culture of a group does influence, but does not determine, the way that people live. The cultural heroes and heroines described in both traditional and contemporary stories and songs may support a belief that pain and suffering and death should be borne with stoicism, and such a tradition may have been developed by both the experience of hard working conditions and child-rearing practices which prepared people for those conditions. In a different way, a culture may influence people by creating ideas about what is appropriate behaviour for women, how to respond to the pains of the menstrual cycle, for example (van den Akker *et al.* 1995), or by providing them with ideas about some foods being suitable only for men or for women. It may also provide them with ideas about their appearance and body shape, and all of these influences may affect how they respond to illness and to medical ideas about treatment, particularly when the treatment involves diet. Detailing such differences and the beliefs that they are based on may, if it is well done, help to break down crude stereotypical views of ethnic minority groups and show that the behaviours which health professionals and others find hard to understand are based on values and beliefs, not just ignorance of the English way of life. Hammersley (1995), in writing about the politics of anti-racism, accepts the view that research may in many cases do no more than attempt to correct common-sense assumptions. But this limited objective may be of real value if the findings of culturally based research are disseminated in ways which can influence practice. There is validity in the criticisms of culturally based research made by Donovan (1986) and others that it tends to concentrate on 'the exotic and unusual' and to identify the cultural practices of minority groups which are seen as harmful to their health, but many of the studies quoted are early ones and it is surely less true now to say that 'The aim is to change the people to match existing services, rather than altering services to meet people's perceived needs' (Donovan 1986: 47).

Studies such as the 1952 Zborowski study of cultural differences in response to pain may well have contributed to the stereotypical views held by health care professionals and also contributed to prejudices which suggest that people in some groups are always complainers and their requests for more painkillers can be ignored (Bowler 1993). But they also alerted us to what appears to be a real problem of how a culture shapes people's responses to pain. A more sophisticated understanding of how culture may influence responses to pain is dependent on such beginnings. This entails getting rid of the essentialist view of ethnicity, which suggests that all people from a particular ethnic group are essentially the same, and instead recognising that people from any ethnic background will have a number of structures giving relevance to their lives, with their culture and ethnicity being only one such structure which people utilise in making decisions about how to live and how to cope with the problems of illness.

RESEARCH METHOD

The justification for continuing to use the concepts of culture and ethnicity rests on two grounds: first, on the argument that any analysis which does not pay regard to these concepts neglects the important role that they play in showing how individuals and groups construct their identities; second, on practical grounds it is argued that people's perceptions of health and illness are influenced by the taken-for-granted ideas of their culture, as well as by the medical/ scientific knowledge they are able to draw on through their engagement with education, the mass media and the health care system. How individuals respond to the threat of illness, the experience of illness and the treatment regimens is therefore affected by all of these. Ethnographic studies of the living, changing culture of particular ethnic groups will help us to understand their behaviour and to shape our own accordingly. Whilst epidemiological research may show higher rates for particular illnesses or conditions linked to particular ethnic groups, it is not necessarily the case that 'culture' is the 'pathogen'. The low rates of hypertension in some cultural groups (Levin 1994) are evidence of the possible protective effects of cultural membership. Sociological research is more often concerned to show how illness is understood and experienced by a particular ethnic group. This ethnographical approach which is usually adopted by researchers uses culture as a descriptive and analytic concept aiming to produce what Geertz (1993) has called 'thick description', which allows the people in the ethnic group to be heard. It is important that the description is accurate and Hammersley (1995) argues that 'The overriding concern of researchers is the truth of claims, not the political implications or consequences' (Hammersley 1995: 76).

How research is carried out is also important, but in the case of research into the culture of an ethnic minority where the interpretation of behaviour and talk is more than usually problematic, there is an argument for saying that members of that group should be involved in the research. Some (for example, Ahmad 1993) argue that, while they would not exclude white researchers from research concerning black people, black researchers or researchers from the same ethnic background are more likely to be able to be able to get inside the 'skins' of the people to provide an accurate description of the views of that group. Andersen (1993) quotes from Blauner and Wellman (1973) to illustrate this point:

> There are certain aspects of racial phenomena, however, that are particularly difficult, if not impossible, for a member of the oppressing group to grasp empirically and formulate conceptually. These barriers are existential and methodological as well as political and ethical.
>
> (Blauner and Wellman 1973: 329)

Although there are good reasons for encouraging black researchers to research their own communities, one reason being that they might be better able to gain both physical and psychological access to people, there are a number of reasons why such matching of researchers to respondents is not necessarily a good idea. First, it might increase the tendency to use black researchers only for research to do with black communities, thus marginalising them. Second, there are other important markers of identity besides ethnicity or being black or white. Phoenix (1995) makes this point and takes the view that matching interviewers and respondents does not necessarily lead to 'better' data. She is inclined to take the view that 'race' may be more significant in an interview situation than gender, but she also warns that:

> It is, therefore, important to recognise differences and commonalities between people who are socially constructed as belonging to the same group as well as across groups.
>
> (Phoenix 1995: 70)

Rhodes (1994) comes to a similar conclusion. Song (female) and Parker (male) (1995), both of mixed descent, also discuss the complexities of gender and cultural identity in the interview situation in their studies of young Chinese people in England, and argue that whether respondents feel 'commonality or difference' according to gender or cultural identity may fluctuate during the course of one interview. A third reason for arguing against the necessity of matching the ethnic background of researchers with those they are researching is that it appeals to a notion of essentialism, the idea that there are essential differences between people which always override other aspects of their being. The constructionist view of ethnicity which has been developed in this chapter has argued against such an essentialist position.

There are arguments for including people from ethnic minority groups in research teams whether the research is qualitative or quantitative and whether the research is to do with ethnic minorities or not, but these are to do with, in the first case, making equality of opportunity more of a reality. Second, having a team of researchers from varying backgrounds means that different questions may be asked and different interpretations considered, and a more sensitive understanding achieved. Although a researcher may not be from the same ethnic background as the group being studied, he or she may have had experiences of discrimination or may simply have a different perspective which will provoke discussion and the search for the clarification of meaning by the research team. The argument made here is that ethnographic research looking at particular ethnic groups can be justified. Looking into the ways of perceiving and managing health and illness and the cultural significance of cooking and eating particular foods that those groups have, and concentrating on specific groups, can reveal differences within the groups as well as differences between them and other groups. The knowledge gained can also help to breakdown the crude stereotypes that health professionals and others may be working with, and these are strong considerations.

CONCLUSION

This chapter is based on the view that there is both structure and agency in social life and that to ignore agency is as limiting as ignoring structure. The argument for the continuing use of the terms 'ethnicity' and 'culture in health research is based on the view that, although locating people within their ethnic group will not provide a complete explanation of their behaviour, it does give an indication of how they may see themselves as well as how they are constructed as members of political groupings. At a practical level, it may also indicate how they are responding to illness and what they may see as being contributing factors to a healthy life.

What has been stressed in this chapter is the positive way that ordinary people use their understanding of ethnicity in placing themselves in relation to others. The construction of ethnicity is not a one-way process of the state classifying people into ethnic categories as part of a surveillance procedure; it is also a structure of relevance and a process that individuals engage in in order to give meaning to their experiences in life. It is also a process that groups of people use to stake a claim for the resources provided by the state.

In a similar way it has been argued that people selectively draw on elements in the culture of their group to help them manage the situations they face. For some this may mean that, faced with a relative abundance of food, they decide what to buy and what to eat by reference to cultural and religious ideas. Rice crispies are okay, they are not haram (proscribed), so they can be eaten, but a proper meal must have rice in it and be halal. Bangladeshi people in East London go to the supermarket for some goods and to the local shop for things like meat, where the halal/haram distinction is important.

Recognising the importance of ethnicity and culture in people's lives does not deny that the experience of racism is real and threatening, nor that resources and life chances are unequally distributed; but people do find a sense of support from seeing themselves as part of a community, real or imagined. It is not necessarily politically desirable that people are inclined to seek security in 'tribalism', but it is clear that community does give a sense of belonging and a basis for an identity.

Social research can help by identifying what people see as their problems and what they see as relevant in the day-to-day management of their lives and contextualising these within the political and economic structures which shape these lives.

ACKNOWLEDGEMENT

I am grateful to Jonathan Gabe for his comments on an earlier draft of this chapter.

REFERENCES

Ahmad, W. (1993) 'Making black people sick: "race", ideology and health research' in W. Ahmad (ed.) *'Race' and Health in Contemporary Britain*. Buckingham: Open University Press.

Ahmad, W. and Sheldon, T. (1992) 'Race and Statistics' in W. Ahmad (ed.) *The Politics of 'Race' and Health*. Bradford: Race Relations Policy Research Unit, University of Bradford.

van den Akker, O. B. A., Eves, F. F., Service, S. and Lennon, B. (1995) 'Menstrual cycle symptom reporting in three British ethnic groups', *Social Science and Medicine* 40 (10): 1417–1423.

Anderson, B. (1983) *Imagined Communities: Reflections on the Spread of Nationalism*. London: Verso.

Andersen, M. (1993) 'Studying across difference' in J. Stanfield and R. Dennis (eds) *Race and Ethnicity in Research Methods*. London: Sage.

Bagley, C. and Binitie, A. (1970) 'Alcoholism and schizophrenia in Irishmen in London,' *British Journal of Addiction* 65: 3–7.

Barth, F. (1969) *Ethnic Groups and Boundaries*, London: George Allen & Unwin.

Bauman, Z. (1992) *Intimations of Postmodernity*. London: Routledge.

Bhabba, H. (1994) *The Location of Culture*. London: Routledge.

Bhrolchain, M. (1990) 'The ethnicity question for the 1991 census: background and issues,' *Ethnic and Racial Studies* 13 (4): 244–246.

Blauner, R. & Wellman, D. (1973) 'Towards the de-colonization of social research,' quoted in M. Andersen (1993) 'Studying across difference' in J. Stanfield and R. Dennis (eds) *Race & Ethnicity in Research Methods*. London: Sage.

Bowler, I. (1993) 'They're not the same as us: midwives stereotypes of South Asian descent maternity patients,' *Sociology of Health and Illness*, 15 (2): 157–178.

Brah, A. (1992) 'Difference, diversity and differentiation' in J. Donald and A. Rattansi (eds) *Race, Culture and Difference*. London: Sage.

Brah, A. (1994) 'Time, place, & others: discourses of race, nation and ethnicity', *Sociology* 28 (3): 805–813.

British Medical Association (1995) *Multicultural Health Care*. London: British Medical Association.

Centre for Bangladeshi Studies (1994) *Routes and Beyond*. London: Centre for Bangladeshi Studies.

Directorate of Public Health, East London & City Health Authority *Annual Report (1995/6)*. London: HMSO.

Donovan, J. (1986) *We Don't Buy Sickness. It Just Comes*. Aldershot: Gower Press.

Fanon, F. (1986) *Black Skin, White Masks*. London: Pluto.

Garfinkel, H. (1984) *Studies in Ethnomethodology*. Cambridge: Polity Press.

Geertz, C. (1993) *The Interpretation of Cultures*. London: Fontana

Goldberg, D. (1993) *Racist Culture*. Oxford: Blackwell.

Hall, S. (1992a) 'The question of cultural identity' in S. Hall, D. Held and A. McGrew *Modernity and its Futures*. Cambridge: Polity Press.

Hall, S. (1992b) 'New ethnicities' in J. Donald and A. Rattansi (eds) *Race, Culture and Difference*. London: Sage.

Hammersley, M. (1995) *The Politics of Social Research*. London: Sage.

Kushnick, L. (1988) 'Racism, the National Health Service, and the health of black people,' *International Journal of Health Services* 18 (3): 457–470.

Levin, J. (1994) *Religion in Aging and Health*. London: Sage.

McKenzie, K. & Crowcroft, N. (1994) 'Race, ethnicity, culture and science,' *British Medical Journal* 309: 286–287.

Modood, T. (1994) 'Political Blackness and British Asians,' *Sociology* 28 (4): 859–876.

Modood, T., Beishon, S. and Virdee, S. (eds) (1994) *Changing Ethnic Identities*. London: Policy Studies Institute.

Nagel, J. (1994) 'Constructing ethnicity: creating and recreating ethnic identity & culture,' *Social Problems* 41 (1): 152–176.

Pearson, M. (1983) 'The politics of ethnic minority health studies', *Radical Community Medicine* 16: 34–44.

Perkins, K. (1994) 'Elderly Irish – A Forgotten Minority? Making the case for culturally sensitive services', London Guildhall University, unpublished M.Sc. dissertation.

Phoenix, A. (1995) 'Practising feminist research: the intersection of gender and "race" in the research process?' in M. Maynard and J. Purvis (eds) *Researching Women's Lives from a Feminist Perspective*. London: Taylor & Francis.

Raftery, J., Jones, D. and Rosato, M. (1990) 'The mortality of first and second generation Irish immigrants in the UK' *Social Science and Medicine* 31 (5): 577–584.

Rattansi, A. (1992) 'Racism, culture and education' in J. Donald and A. Rattansi (eds) *Race, Culture and Difference*. London: Sage.

Rex, J. (1986) 'The Role of class analysis in the study of race relations – a Weberian perspective' in J. Rex and D. Mason (eds) *Theories of Race and Ethnic Relations*. Cambridge: Cambridge University Press.

Rhodes, P. (1994) 'Race of interviewer effects in qualitative research: a brief comment', *Sociology* 28 (2): 547–558.

Sashidharan, S. and Francis, E. (1993) 'Epidemiology, ethnicity and schizophrenia' in A. Ahmad (ed.) *Race and Health in Contemporary Britain*. Buckingham: Open University Press.

Schutz, A. (1966) 'Some structures of the life-world' in T. Luckmann (ed.) *Phenomenology and Sociology*. London: Pengiun.

Senior, P. and Bhopal, R. (1994) 'Ethnicity as a variable in epidemiological research', *British Medical Journal* 309: 326–329.

Smaje, C. (1995) *Health, Race and Ethnicity*. London: King's Fund Institute.

Song, M. and Parker, D. (1995) 'Cultural identity: disclosing commonality and difference in in-depth interviewing', *Sociology* 29: 2.

Wallman, S. (1986) 'Ethnicity and the boundary process in context', in J. Rex and D. Mason (eds) *Theories of Race and Ethnic Relations*. Cambridge: Cambridge University Press.

Weber, M. (1968) *Economy and Society*. New York: Bedminster Press.

Zborowski, M. (1952) 'Cultural components in responses to pain', *Journal of Social Issues* 8: 16–30.

Chapter 5

Afro-Caribbean lay beliefs about diabetes
An exploratory study

Mary Pierce and David Armstrong

Diabetes mellitus is a disease of carbohydrate metabolism character-ised by abnormally high blood sugar. People with diabetes live on average 10 years less than those without the disease. It causes blind-ness, renal failure, peripheral vascular disease leading to gangrene and is a significant risk factor for cardiovascular disease. Diabetes is now the leading cause of blindness in the UK; it is the commonest cause of end-stage renal failure, and more than one in two patients with diabetes die early of heart disease or stroke.

Since the discovery and isolation of insulin, dramatic improve-ments have been made in the prognosis of the disease for those patients, usually children, whose own insulin production ceases. However, most patients with diabetes (about nine out of ten cases) maintain some insulin production and need treating with diet and drugs to boost their insulin output. Because they do not require insulin, these latter patients are usually labelled as having non-insulin-dependent diabetes mellitus (NIDDM).

Diabetes is a particular problem for Afro-Caribbean people living in the UK, for two reasons. The first is that rates of diabetes are very high in this population (Cruickshank *et al.* 1990; McKeigue, Shah and Marmot 1991), reflecting the high prevalence of the dis-ease in the Caribbean. The estimated prevalence of diabetes in the Caribbean ranges from 2 per cent to 6 per cent. There are probably about 600,000 people with diabetes in the area, with women being affected twice as often as men. The prevalence rates in the under-30 age group are low and rise to a peak in the sixth decade. In Trinidad 20 per cent of the middle-aged population has been found to have NIDDM (Beckles *et al.* 1986). Diabetes is a leading cause of death in Jamaica (Alleyne *et al.* 1989).

The second reason why diabetes is a particular problem for the

Afro-Caribbean population is the importance of patients' beliefs about diabetes and their effect on health-related behaviours. The successful management of diabetes depends on patients making radical alterations to their lifestyle in terms of changing their diet, losing weight, taking up exercise, taking daily medication in the form of tablets or injections, and regularly attending follow-up appointments. These demands pose problems enough for any population, as is evidenced by the fact that diabetic care is centred on the education of the person with diabetes and support for him or her in making and monitoring these changes (McKinnon 1994). These problems are likely to be compounded for Afro-Caribbean people in the UK as they have cultural beliefs, especially about diet and body shape, that make it even more difficult or perhaps impossible to make changes recommended by professional carers usually more attuned to the beliefs of the dominant white culture.

Although there has been some work looking specifically at Asians' beliefs about diabetes (Kelleher and Islam 1994), there has been no previous work on Afro-Caribbean lay beliefs about diabetes and its management. Other studies that have looked at Afro-Caribbean beliefs have shown marked cultural differences compared with white populations (Morgan and Watkins 1988; Thorogood 1988). It therefore seemed fruitful to begin to explore Afro-Caribbean beliefs about diabetes.

As so little is known about the sorts of problems and perspectives that characterise Afro-Caribbean people's experience of diabetes, a qualitative methodology was judged as particularly appropriate so as not to contaminate their responses with the specific question-and-response sets of the more common structured questionnaire. It was decided to use group interviews to obtain these ideas, in part because it offered an efficient means of obtaining the views of a number of people. In addition, it was felt that the 'discussion' element that accompanies a group interview could be important in eliciting the views held by this ethnic group. The object of the interviews was not to identify the 'typical' Afro-Caribbean view of diabetes, but rather the range of perspectives that characterise Afro-Caribbean people's experience of diabetes.

THE FOCUS GROUPS METHOD

Focus groups developed out of work on the effect on audiences of mass media campaigns during the 1940s and 1950s (Merton,

Fiske and Curtis 1946; Merton, Fiske and Kendall 1956) and have since been used extensively in market research, programme evaluation and public policy settings. The technique has also been used increasingly in health services research in the USA (e.g., Multiple Risk Factor Intervention Trial Group 1982). Focus groups are now increasingly used as an exploratory instrument or to illuminate earlier quantitative results (Reynolds and Johnson 1978).

Focus groups usually consist of 8 to 12 members under the direction of a moderator. The term 'focus' refers to the role of the moderator in limiting discussion to areas of interest. Verbal and non-verbal information can be gathered, and responses may be elaborated, defended or criticised by other members, producing ideas that may have been missed in individual settings.

While the Afro-Caribbean patients attending a diabetic clinic could have provided the members of a focus group, it was felt that such a method of obtaining the group might place too much of a 'medical' framework on subsequent discussion. Besides, it was likely that many patients would choose not to use the clinic precisely as a result of their particular beliefs about diabetes. Accordingly, it seemed more appropriate to identify a more 'community' sample. Brixton Neighbourhood Community Association met this purpose. It is a community group providing a social centre for mainly older Afro-Caribbean people in Brixton. Officers of the Association reported a large number of their members as having diabetes and being willing to come and discuss their illness.

Two group interviews were carried out at the Association's local offices: there were nine people in the first group and eight in the second. Most of the interviewees were over 65 years of age and the majority were male. A number of open questions and 'prompts' about the experience of diabetes were drawn up and used to guide the discussion. The questions enquired about the everyday experience and understanding of diabetes and also views about the available professional care. Each of the two interviews lasted just over an hour. During both interviews detailed notes were kept by the authors, and these were reviewed immediately after the session. The first interview was actually taped, but background noise in the Association's offices meant that the tape was not useable. The results reported below are based on the two sets of field notes.

WHAT IS DIABETES?

The label of 'diabetic' is given to patients by doctors. For many patients diabetes is symptomless and the disease is diagnosed on the basis of a chance screening of urine. From the presence of sugar in the urine and later confirmatory blood tests doctors can be sure whether or not the disease exists in a certain patient; but for those labelled as 'diabetic', especially if there are no obvious symptoms that can be related to the disease, the nature of the illness and its relationship to the patient is much less clear.

All members of the groups had been invited on the basis that they had diabetes, but not all were certain that they had it. Three respondents in the second group said they did not have diabetes but were 'interested' in it as they knew people with the problem. One respondent reported having an ulcer, though it was not clear whether he directly linked this to diabetes. Another reported that while he had some symptoms of diabetes which were being treated, no doctor had informed him specifically that he was a diabetic. Yet another reported having had diabetes, but now, with his weight under control, he was 'all right'.

The difficulty in determining who considered themselves as having the disease was further complicated by the meaning given to the term, even by those who had received a specific medical diagnosis. For many respondents in the first group, the illness of diabetes seemed entwined with the related problem of having 'sugar'. There seemed some uncertainty as to whether diabetes and 'sugar' were two separate illnesses or all part of the same one. One respondent said that he had been told by his doctor that he had 'sugar' and diabetes, thus affirming for him the distinctiveness of the two illnesses. The distinction made sense to some of them as the relationship between diabetes and 'sugar' seemed to relate to their experiences of the West Indies, where 'sugar' was believed to be rare and diabetes common. In the second focus group no mention was made of 'sugar' as a separate illness and, when challenged, group members said that diabetes and 'sugar' were 'the same thing'. Even so, for them, diabetes was not a 'disease' (this word was reserved for illnesses with an infective, and presumably contagious basis) but an 'ailment': 'sugar' was the 'situation in blood and urine'.

The importance of sugar in relation to diabetes was discussed by both groups. The level of sugar in the blood was held to be important, but group members were confused about how diabetes sometimes seemed to produce high blood sugar and sometimes low. This was compounded by the fact that though the illness was linked to excess sugar, sugar (kept as a sweet in the pocket) was also an important part of therapy. Thus, diabetes was represented as a problem over the body's control of sugar, not as one of high sugar *per se*.

For individual group members, the role of sugar in diabetes was similarly cloudy: one respondent reported that sometimes he had sugar in his urine and sometimes not, but he was never sure why this was so as he could not relate it to his own behaviour. He went on to acknowledge that it could be due to 'sweets or something . . . it's tempting to eat something you shouldn't eat'. Another respondent reported being told by her GP that diabetes was due to 'one part of the ovaries breaking down and being unable to handle sugar'. Another commented that sugar had never been found in his urine, only in his blood, and this 'had led to a belly full of water'. There seemed agreement that having excess sugar intake produced diabetes. However, this did not seem the full story, as they reported evidence from the West Indies that those working with sugar and having a high sugar intake did not have the same problems as in the UK – though this view may have represented some confusion in the group between the apparently two separate illnesses of 'sugar' and diabetes.

The symptoms of diabetes were also believed to be implicated in its causation. Several respondents mentioned drinking a lot of water which in turn contributed to weight gain which then produced diabetes. Overall, it was apparent that respondents' individual experiences were of paramount importance in evaluating evidence about the cause of their illness. For example, one respondent reported himself as confused about the role of weight gain in diabetes because 'some gain weight and some lose weight'. Another, female, respondent thought that depression was a contributory factor in getting diabetes. This view was immediately challenged by someone else who reported that though he never got depressed he still had diabetes.

There was wide agreement in the first group on the issue of whether or nor diabetes ran in families: from the evidence of their own experience only one person could identify someone in their family – in this case a cousin – who had diabetes. However, the second group could identify many more relatives with the illness and agreed that it did run in families. This view was tempered by the mystery of why some got it and others did not. One respondent thought that his children were not at risk as his wife developed the illness after childbearing.

WHAT IS THE EFFECT OF DIABETES?

Not many of the respondents could identify health problems that had emerged as a direct consequence of having diabetes. Some reported that diabetes made them feel weak 'when they had it'. Others mentioned excess drinking, as well as 'eyes getting bad'. However, for almost all the respondents, the experience of diabetes was intimately bound up with their diet. Diabetes was described as an illness which 'burns up quickly what you eat'; this led to incessant hunger, constant eating and weight gain. Nevertheless, weight gain was not simply related to diabetes, as some people gained weight while others lost it (one respondent described her futile attempts to gain weight). In fact, weight gain seemed to be less related to eating habits and more to do with being 'born that way'.

The question of an appropriate diet in diabetes led to a wide-ranging discussion. One respondent thought that the important thing about diet was not to put on too much weight; he had followed this advice and now it seemed that his diabetes was not a problem. The simple medical injunction of 'don't eat' was ridiculed as this might mean not getting the 'right food'. Diet sheets were not held in great respect: one respondent said 'I just threw it away'. Others had been given special diets but chose to go on as usual. Details of the diets that they had been recommended, in particular their paucity, were exchanged – to general laughter. The overall philosophy seemed to be simple: that eating was important for living and changing eating patterns with the apparent object of improving life was contradictory. If anything there was a philosophy of moderation. So long as not too much was eaten then any particular food could be taken, though this seemed to apply particularly to West Indian food. Indeed, for some there was a belief that it may have been English food that contributed to diabetes.

In the second group, there was some recognition that 'starchy' foods were bad. Starchy foods could be identified by where they came from: foods from underground, such as potatoes and yams, were believed to be very starchy, whereas those from above ground, such as bananas and plantain, were not. The effect of starchy foods seemed to be strongly mediated by the weather. In the West Indies, a lot of starchy foods were eaten, but the hot sun and general heat ensured that these foods were 'burned up'. Perspiration then got rid of the toxins produced by the burning up of the food. Thus, it was the failure to perspire sufficiently in the UK that made starchy foods into a potentially dangerous factor. One example was quoted – to general approval – of someone with diabetes returning to the West Indies, where their diabetes cleared up, only for it to reappear on their return to the UK. Further corroboration was provided by another respondent who had worked in a bakery in Britain where he regularly perspired: it was only after he stopped working there that he developed diabetes.

IS DIABETES A SERIOUS ILLNESS?

There was general agreement that diabetes was a serious illness and that someone with the disease would never get better and never be cured. However, if diet was taken properly then this would lead to a normal life. Without treatment it was reported that one would die earlier 'from too much sugar'. The first group could not think of any medical consequences of diabetes, though the second identified comas, strokes and heart attacks. Both groups also discussed the dangers of getting cuts – which could lead to the loss of an arm or leg. Reflecting the strong views they had on diet there was laughter when it was pointed out that 'the dietician will kill you'.

Despite identifying 'keeping diabetes under control' as the treatment ideal, their day-to-day priorities seemed to interfere with this. The value of diets was acknowledged: 'it has been said that it can be controlled by diet – but that diet is very strict', but changing eating patterns was another matter. 'You must eat wisely, but sometimes eat foolishly' was a comment with which most seemed to concur. Diabetes seemed to disturb a long-term pattern of eating, and these respondents seemed to have difficulty in establishing another pattern which could be stable over time.

One respondent – one of only two on insulin – reported skipping her medication on some days as she 'got fed up with it'. She also said that when her sister developed insulin-dependent diabetes she said to herself that she would rather die than take those injections; in the event she had to follow her sister, but she had managed to adjust to it. Most respondents agreed that they would not like insulin. One said that she was scared of needles ('I'm allergic to them') and that this motivated her to watch her weight and avoid needing insulin. It was observed that taking insulin was a sort of dependency because 'once you've started you can never come off'.

THE GP OR HOSPITAL?

The view of the respective spheres of influence of general practice and hospital was that the latter treated the more serious aspects of the illness. Thus, it was felt that their GP would refer them to hospital if the illness was harder to treat or medication needed changing. The corollary of this was that patients attending hospital for their diabetes had a more serious form of the disease or were more difficult to treat.

Over all, the treatment obtained from both GPs and hospital was praised. However, there was some discussion about the quality of explanations given by doctors. On the one hand, it was pointed out that doctors always reported whether the blood sugar was high or low but, on the other hand, doctors did not seem to tell much about the illness itself. One respondent pointed out that nurses could not be a source of explanation as they did not know enough about the illness to explain anything of value.

Finally, on the question of possible improvements to the care they received from the health service, none of the respondents could identify any specific changes that they would like to see in either the general practice or hospital care they received. What they would have liked ideally was a 'cure' for their illness, but they recognised that this was not possible at the moment – though one person thought he had heard that there was 'something in the pipeline which will help diabetes in future'. As one respondent reported, 'the pancreas is dead, it cannot pass out sugar; it keeps piling up'.

INDIVIDUAL DIFFERENCES, LAY CULTURE AND WEST INDIAN CULTURE

This exploratory study identified a number of important beliefs about diabetes and its management held by these respondents. Given the significant differences between these accounts and conventional medical explanations of diabetes, it would seem appropriate to label these views as 'lay beliefs'. Without interviewing corresponding groups of non Afro-Caribbeans it is more difficult to say whether these accounts also represented examples of 'ethnic beliefs'. Nevertheless, a number of views were expressed that clearly did seem to reflect a specific and different ethnic culture.

First, views about the relative merits of Afro-Caribbean food versus English food, and the concept of 'ideal' body size seemed heavily influenced by Afro-Caribbean cultural beliefs. Second, the role of sweating and heat in the development of diabetes in relationship to the experience of sugar-cane cutting is linked to the Afro-Caribbean experience and embedded in that culture. And third, ideas about the relationship of migration to England in the aetiology of diabetes may be related to personal experience of migration or part of Afro-Caribbean cultural beliefs – though it may be a belief held more widely by migrant groups other than those from the Caribbean.

On the other hand, somewhat surprisingly, no mention was made by any of the groups of the use of folk remedies, such as fenugreek, annatto or karella. This is in marked contrast to the extensive use of folk remedies described by Donovan in her study of people of Afro-Caribbean origin living in London (Donovan 1986). It is possible that these remedies are not used for specific diseases such as diabetes, being more usually taken for symptoms. Yet this would be ironic, as certain West-Indian medicinal plants are known to have quite specific beneficial effects in diabetes. Indeed, the World Health Organisation, is actively promoting research into the abstracts of indigenous plants that folklore considers helpful for diabetes (Morrison and West 1982, 1985). Alternatively, as discussed below, the two investigators may have constrained the groups' willingness to discuss these issues.

ISSUES OF METHOD

The focus group methodology seemed to work well. First, like any qualitative methodology, it allows exploration of themes less hampered by the investigators' own agenda than is the case in a more structured questionnaire survey. But, in addition, it also proved a very economical way of investigating the views of a relatively large number of subjects in a short time. Second, because the discussion ranged fairly freely within the group, a number of issues emerged that might not have been revealed in a one-to-one interview. For example, the willingness to lampoon doctors' and dietitians' instructions on diet was aided by the sharing of stories and the responsive laughter that accompanied them. Third, many of the attempts at clarification or challenging of statements came from the group itself (though often as an attempt to advance an alternative view or experience).

There are several recognised problems with group interviews. They include a risk that the group process may be dominated by certain members and that people who are more shy may feel unable to express their views, particularly if they feel they might be challenged. It is also more difficult in a focus group to explore an individual's opinions without disrupting the flow of conversation in the group, in contrast to individual interviews, where in-depth investigation is more feasible. However, none of these potential difficulties seemed to be a major problem in this study; the problems that were experienced were general to the methodology but seemed particularly acute in this study.

Tape recording a discussion among a number of people is inherently more difficult in a group compared to a one-to-one interview. Besides the technical problems of picking up all voices clearly, there is a greater tendency for one speaker to overlap with another. This can produce particular problems for transcribing, especially if an attempt is made to identify individual speakers. These problems were compounded in this study by the background noise that ultimately made the tapes impossible to use (though the advantages of meeting the groups on their own territory and the relaxed approach that it engendered probably counterbalanced the loss of a taped record).

The second problem that was encountered was the occasional question from the group to the facilitators on some technical aspect of diabetes. This is a problem for any interview that seeks to establish 'lay views', in that this presumes a pre-existing 'expert view'. As is well established, people can hold both 'public' and 'private' views on a subject and may seek to clarify or seek support for the former during an interview (Cornwall 1984). This problem was particularly important in this study as both moderators (DA and MP) were medically qualified and had announced at the beginning of the session that they were from a medical school/hospital. Thus, respondents would sometimes ask for the 'expert view' on some aspect of their diabetes or for an adjudication on some dispute within the group. It was felt inappropriate to try and answer these questions at this time, so a number of strategies were deployed to avoid doing so. Sometimes interviewees' questions were deflected by asking for their own views on the topic or by trying to change the subject. More persistent questioning was met by a 'minimalist' response. All these strategies, however, seemed awkward and felt like an ungenerous way of treating people who were so willing to help with the study. Whether or not the fear that an 'expert view' would in fact have undermined the wide-ranging discussion that occurred in the groups was never really tested, but perhaps this is a particular problem for 'experts' running groups or carrying out interviews.

The use of 'experts' as group facilitators may also have inhibited discussion of some topics. This may account for the lack of mention of folk remedies for diabetes, though the group seemed willing to voice many 'unconventional' views on other topics. Perhaps these particular individuals do not use folk remedies, or perhaps in the last decade their usage has decreased significantly.

IMPLICATIONS

Often, during the interviews, there was a sense that reports of conversations with doctors were a pale shadow of what they actually had been told in hospital; but once they had had time to discuss the problems amongst themselves it was apparent that views about diabetes were embedded in much deeper-seated cultural beliefs about health and illness. All of these patients have been 'told', probably on numerous occasions, about their diabetes, but they had failed to 'learn'. This failure was often not conductive for the best long-term management of what can be a seriously debilitating disease. But, if education is the answer, it is not to an 'ignorant' population but to one that is surprisingly knowledgeable and sophisticated in views about diabetes, though these views might not equate with those of their professional carers. This presents a challenge to 'diabetic educators': is it these patients or the health professionals who need to change their beliefs?

This exploratory study has raised as many questions as it answered. There is a need to explore further the views of Afro-Caribbean people about their diabetes so that their current behaviour can better be understood in a sensitive way. Furthermore, it is necessary to see to what extent these views are unique to the Afro-Caribbean population. Finally, what this study did show was that a focus group methodology could be used successfully in this type of investigation, particularly in its mechanism for allowing the discussion and verbalisation of cultural beliefs.

REFERENCES

Alleyne, S. A., Cruickshank, J. K., Golding, A. L. and Morrison, E. Y. St. A. (1989) 'Mortality from diabetes in Jamaica,' *Bulletin of Pan American Health Organization* 23: 306–15

Basch, C. (1987) 'Focus group interview: an under-utilised research technique for improving theory and practice in health education', *Health Education Quarterly*; 14 (4): 411–448.

Beckles, G. L. A., Miller G. J., Kirkwood, B. *et al.* (1986) 'High total and cardiovascular mortality in adults of Indian descent in Trinidad not explained by major coronary risk factors,' *Lancet* 1: 1298–1301.

Cornwall, J. (1984) *Hard-earned Lives*. Tavistock: London.

Cruickshank, J. K., Cooper, J., Macduff, J. and Drubra, U. (1990) 'Glucose tolerance in N-W London: the prevalence and inheritance of diabetes by ethnic group with suggestions for prevention,' *Diabetic Medicine* 7 (supplement 2): 52.

Donovan, J. (1986) *We Don't Buy Sickness, It Just Comes*. Aldershot: Gower.

Kelleher, D. and Islam, S. (1994) 'The problem of integration: Asian people and diabetes,' *Journal of the Royal Society of Medicine* 87: 414–417.

McKeigue, P. M., Shah, B. and Marmot M. G. (1991) 'Relation of central obesity and insulin resistance with high diabetes prevalence and cardiovascular risk in South Asians,' *Lancet* 337: 382–386.

McKinnon, M. (1994) *Providing Diabetes Care in General Practice*. London: Class Publishing.

Merton, R. K., Fiske, M. and Curtis, C. (1946) *Mass Persuasion*. New York: Harper & Row.

Merton, R. K., Fiske, M. and Kendall P. L. (1956) *The Focused Interview*. New York: Free Press.

Morgan, M. and Watkins, C. J. (1988) 'Managing hypertension: beliefs and responses to medication among cultural groups,' *Sociology of Health and Illness* 10 (4): 561–578.

Morrison, E. Y. St A. and West, M. A. (1982) 'A preliminary study of the effect of some West-Indian Medicinal Plants on blood sugar levels in the dog,' *West Indian Medical Journal* 31: 194–197.

Morrison, E. Y. St A. and West, M. A. (1985) 'The effects of Bixella orellano (annatto) on blood sugar levels in the anesthetised dog,' *West Indian Medical Journal* 34: 38–42.

Multiple Risk Factor Intervention Trial Group (1982) 'Multiple Risk factor intervention trial: risk factors changes and mortality results,' *JAMA* 248: 1465–1477.

Reynolds, F. D. and Johnson, D. K. (1978) 'Validity of focus group findings,' *Journal of Advertising Research* 18: 21–24.

Thorogood, N. (1988) 'Health and management of daily lives among females of Afro-Caribbean origin living in Hackney,' University of London unpublished Ph.D. thesis.

Chapter 6

The health of the Irish in England

David Kelleher and Sheila Hillier

INTRODUCTION

A study of the health of the Irish in England illustrates nicely the methodological and conceptual difficulties involved in explaining differences in the health status of immigrant groups and the 'host' population. A number of studies (Greenslade 1992; Williams 1992) have considered aspects of the health of Irish people in England and this chapter is an attempt to develop the analysis. The question explored is based on the available empirical evidence about the health and illness behaviour of the Irish in England. Although the statistical data presented is by no means conclusive, and indeed is open to question on a number of counts, it could be said to be pointing to the conclusion that the health of Irish people in England remains poorer than that of English people. The question of whether this 'social fact' can be explained by showing that many Irish immigrants can be found in social classes 4 and 5 is discussed and the alternative explanation that Irish immigrants may be in poor health before they emigrate to England is also considered. The suggestion that the average health of the Irish in England is made to appear poor because of the existence of a minority who live in hostels or on the streets is another strand which is considered. The economic position of the Irish in England is also discussed. The final section considers the extent to which the poor health of the Irish people in England can be explained by reference to ideas about the culture and identity of Irish people and how these have been shaped by the postcolonial experience and, in particular, the experience of living in the land of the colonial power as an immigrant. The analysis will therefore include political and economic factors and their links with the lived-in culture.

Irish people have been coming to work and live in England in large numbers for nearly 200 years (Jackson 1963), and although their presence has been strongly resented from time to time, many of them have settled and intermarried with the English (Ryan 1990). In some ways they have remained a distinct group, however, different by virtue of their Catholic religion, by the occupations they are associated with (there were 31,000 Irish nurses working in England in 1971 and the 1991 census shows that 32 per cent of Irish men born in the Republic are working in the construction industry) and their tendency to settle in particular parts of large towns such as Liverpool, Manchester and London where they have created an Irish culture. Although often perceived in work situations and in popular culture as different and often inferior to the native English, in government statistics they have either been recorded as English or placed in a residual category as 'white other' with a varied collection of non-black foreigners. When they have appeared as a separate group in government statistics and been shown to have high rates of conviction for crimes such as vagrancy or drunkeness (Ryan 1990) or for having a high rate of mental illness (Cochrane 1983) it has generally been explained that these aspects of the Irish are a result of their low class position. It has been assumed that the high rates were only what could be expected of 'McAlpine's Fusiliers'. For reasons which will be explored later the Irish tended to accept the position they were ascribed, and it is only recently that some Irish people in England have made a case for saying that the Irish have a culture and ethnicity which is distinct from that of the English. The question then arises as to whether elements in that culture can be seen to be useful in explaining the high rates of illness experienced by the Irish in England without pathologising Irish culture. It becomes important to identify the part played by culture and to ask whether there is a sense in which the history of English–Irish relations has contributed to Irish culture a sense of being underdogs, which may in turn emphasise the existing stoicism of Irish immigrants. The part played by material factors which are a result of their class position has also to be considered. That is the task of this book, to raise these substantive and methodological issues for debate. First, though, it is necessary to establish what evidence there is for saying that the Irish in England have poorer health than might be expected from such a long-established immigrant group when the commonly accepted wisdom is that the health of such groups tends to become more like that of the host community than that of the people they left behind. As Raftery, Jones and Rosato (1990) note:

> Migrant studies have often shown that immigrant groups take on the morbidity and mortality patterns of the host community over time.
>
> (Raftery, Jones and Rosato 1990: 578)

THE EVIDENCE

A useful starting-point is to look at the adult and infant mortality rates. The mortality rates for Irish men and women between the ages 20 and 69 living in England and Wales are considerably higher than the rates for the country as a whole. The OPCS Mortality and Geography review in the 1980s reports that:

> Overall mortality varied between country of birth groups . . . There were significantly high levels at ages 20–69 in males from Ireland (SMR 128).
>
> (OPCS 1990: 106)

It continues by saying

> The findings are broadly similar among women, with the highest mortality at ages 20–69 among the Irish (SMR 120).
>
> (ibid.)

The same report shows that at the younger age group of 20–49 the rates were even higher for both men and women, the SMR for men being 147 and for women 123. These mortality rates are higher than the rates for any other immigrant group apart from the rate for African women who, in the 20–49 age group, have an SMR of 127. The OPCS study also notes that by the 1980s the SMR for Irish men had declined relatively little compared with other groups:

> Mortality of immigrants in 1970–72 and 1979–83 showed significant differences between groups in the rate of mortality decline. The greatest improvements were observed for African and Caribbean men and women with mortality falling sharply over the period . . . In contrast, the high mortality among Scottish and Irish showed the least improvement over the decade, and by the 1980s these groups had the highest mortality of the groups examined.
>
> (OPCS 1990: xxi)

While some of this excess of mortality over what might be expected could be linked to the poorer living and working conditions of people in social classes 4 and 5, Marmot, Adelstein and Buluso (1984) show that for Irish men aged 15–64 living in England the SMR is higher than for all men in England and Wales in every social class. The SMR for all men in England and Wales in social class 1 was 77, whereas for Irish men the SMR was 96. At the other end of the social scale, in social class 5, the England and Wales SMR was 137 but the SMR for Irish men was 157.

The infant mortality rate (1982–1985) for children born in England to Irish mothers was higher than that for children born to English mothers, but not markedly so; the English rate being 9.7 per 1,000 live births and the Irish rate 10.1, with the greatest difference being to mothers with three or more children already. The difference here being 11.7 per 1,000 for English mothers and 14.0 for Irish mothers (OPCS 1990), and as the Irish women have a higher fertility rate than the English women they are more likely to be producing children in families where there are already two children. Smaje (1995) presents more details of deaths from specific causes and makes some comparisons with other ethnic groups.

Differences in the causes of death among adults has led to some hypotheses being developed and others challenged (Adelstein *et al.* 1986a; Skrabanek 1986) and these therefore need also to be given some consideration. Adelstein *et al.* (1986a) compare the causes of death of Irish immigrants to the causes of death of Irish people living in Ireland and to the causes of death of English people living in England. After considering a number of possible explanations for the sustained higher SMRs of Irish immigrants, Adelstein and his colleagues conclude that the major causes of death of Irish immigrants all have a behavioural element in them:

> While the all-cause mortality of Irish male immigrants is higher than in Irish males, this disparity between the immigrant figure and the Irish figure is highest in conditions probably determined by behaviour viz. cancer of the buccal cavity and pharynx, of the rectum, of the lung, peptic ulcer and cirrhosis of the liver (smoking and alcohol) and accidents, poisonings and violence.
>
> (Adelstein *et al.* 1986: 189)

A similar argument based on slightly different statistics is made for Irish women. There is also recognition of the fact that many Irish immigrants will have moved from a rural environment to an urban one, but this change of circumstance is seen as less important than the change in behaviour.

Skrabanek (1986) objects to the interpretation that Adelstein and his colleagues place on their statistics. He argues that they have selected their statistics in order to make the case for the importance of behavioural factors. He writes: 'The authors insinuate that the Irish in England do not behave and that they pay for it by death' (Skrabanek 1986: 331). In the same issue of the Irish Medical Journal Adelstein *et al.* (1986a) are given the opportunity to reply to Skrabanek's accusations. They say that using the term 'behaviour' is not synonymous with 'victim blaming' and that their interpretation was legitimate 'speculation'.

In general it appears that the Irish in England die from much the same causes as the English, although Irish-born people are much more likely than the English to die from tuberculosis and slightly more likely to die from external causes (accidents etc.). In the analysis of Marmot, Adelstein and Bulusu (1984) compared to a standardised rate for England and Wales of 100, Irish men in England had a TB rate of 245 and Irish women a rate of 215. Death rates from external causes are given as 180 for men and 135 for women. Raftery *et al.* (1990) also note the high TB rate, high incidence of accidents, poisonings and a high violence rate (external causes) and the relatively high rate in women of neoplasms of the trachea, bronchus and lung, but they argue that as the five main causes of death account for only a small proportion of all deaths, it is not reasonable to attribute the higher SMRs of Irish people in England to any particular cause of death.

Marmot, Adelstein and Bulusu (1984) suggest that some of these rates, for TB for example, are likely to have been influenced by the experience of life in the early years in the country of origin, a point which will be addressed later when a comparison is made between the health of Irish people living in England and those living in Ireland.

Apart from the mortality statistics quoted above there are also some morbidity statistics on the Irish in Britain which should be considered.

The Labour Force Survey (Department of Employment 1993), a sample survey which excludes people living in hostels and therefore excludes a number of Irish construction workers, notes that 20 per cent of the working-age Irish in Britain have health problems or disabilites which limit the work they can do. This compares with 14 per cent for the rest of the population. Data from the 1991 census shows a similar situation, with 17 per cent of Irish-born people stating that they have a long-term illness compared to only 12 per cent of all residents of Britain (table 12, 1991 census report:). For Irish men the figure is 18 per cent compared to 12 per cent for men in Britain as a whole. Owen (1995) notes that some of the excess morbidity can be explained by the age structure of the Irish population in England being skewed to the older age ranges but adds that the rates of illness for Irish-born people are still 5 to 10 per cent higher than expected when age is controlled for. It seems unlikely that many of these people are malingerers, as another set of statistics sheds some light on the illness behaviour and illness experience of Irish people in England. The data from the joint Royal College of General Practitioners (RGCP), OPCS and Department of Health Morbidity Statistics from General Practice (McCormick and Rosenbaum 1990), although only a sample survey of patients in 25 practices, give an indication of what illnesses GPs see people as suffering from and the frequency of their visits to GPs. The Irish, both men and women, visit their GP slightly less than average for England and Wales, having a standardised score of 97 when the average is 100, but they visit more often for what are classified as serious illnesses, Irish men having a score of 117 and Irish women a score of 104. When it comes to illness which is classified as trivial, Irish men visit the doctor less than the average, having a score of 96. Irish women have an average score of 101 for trivial illness.

It is not possible to attach a great deal of significance to differences in morbidity in relation to particular causes of illness, but the rates of attendance at GPs' surgeries for some types of illness may be useful in constructing an analysis at a higher level of generality. First, the rate of attendance of Irish men for neoplasms is 130, but this may well be explained by the low number of such cases in the sample. Two other rates are of interest. The first is the rate of patients registered but not consulting. Here, the Irish are the only identifiable ethnic group with a lower than average rate of consulting, with Irish men having a rate of 107 and Irish women having a rate of 109. The comment on non-consulters is rather obscure and does not mention the Irish, although they seem to fit into several of the categories of non-consulters listed:

Categories of patient apparently most likely not to consult a doctor are the single, those living in non-council rented accommodation, men aged 65 or over who live alone, people of ethnic origin other than the United Kingdom, Caribbean or Indian subcontintent.

(McCormick and Rosenbaum 1990: 34)

The fact that the Irish are less likely than the average person living in the UK to consult a doctor about illness may indicate something relating to their cultural beliefs about health which could be significant in explaining the overall problem of why they have higher mortality rates, but this will be discussed later.

Worthy of comment is the very high rate of consultations for illnesses which are classified as mental disorders. Irish men have a rate of 159, well above the average, and Irish women also have a high rate of 125. This finding gives support to earlier studies of hospital admissions quoted by Cochrane (1983) and discussed by Raftery, Jones and Rosato (1990) and challenges the at first puzzling 1979 study by Cochrane and Stopes-Roe which suggests that the Irish in Britain do not have more mental illness than the native English. This study was a comparative community-based study which compared levels of psychological disturbance rather than mental illness as defined by admissions. The authors discuss why their study produced the unexpected result and suggest that the questionnaire used may not have been sensitive to the symptoms of alcoholism, one of the conditions from which Irish men are frequently said to suffer. The authors also admit that, because of being Irish and living in England, the Irish people might have been unwilling to reveal socially undesirable or incriminating information to outsiders. Another limitation to this study is that, not only did it not include people living in hostels but compared with the English sample it included:

a higher proportion of Irish respondents being in the UK Regis-trar General's classes one and two . . . The English group were also somewhat less likely to own their houses and somewhat more likely to be council tenants than either the Irish or the immigrant group.

(Cochrane and Stopes-Roe 1979: 307)

These limitations probably explain the difference between the find-ings of this study and other studies. As Cochrane (1983) showed, Irish men and women were much more likely to be admitted to hospital for psychiatric treatment than people from any other group when all psychiatric conditions were aggregated (1,054 per 100,000 for men and 1,102 for women as compared with rates of 418 and 583 for English-born people). A later study by Cochrane and Bal (1989) showed that when schizophrenia alone was considered people from the Caribbean had the highest rate, but the Irish had the second highest, and the Irish had the highest rate for all other psychiatric conditions including depression and alcohol abuse. Cochrane (1983) at first noted that these high rates of admission to hospital corresponded with high admission rates in Ireland, which suggested that either genetic or cultural explanations might be appropriate, but a later community-based study in England (Cochrane and Bal 1987) indicated that Irish people living in England had a lower level of mental illness than the native English population. This led Cochrane to repeat his 1979 suggestion that high hospital admission figures could be explained by saying that they included homeless people who would not have been included in the community sample.

Whether the high rates of mental illness can be explained in this way is open to question. Raftery, Jones and Rosato (1990) seem to doubt it, but the study *Alcohol and Disadvantage Amongst the Irish in England* (Harrison and Carr-Hill 1992) does give some support to this hypothesis that the high rates of mental illness found in Irish immigrants can be explained by the inclusion in hospital statistics of a group of homeless and alcoholic people. They say that their analysis of GHS data shows that:

> It is clearly difficult to study such sub-groups comprehensively yet any investigation of the health and social problems facing the Irish in Britain must take account of homelessness.
>
> (Harrison and Carr-Hill 1992: 23)

They go on to say

> The Irish are also the ethnic group most likely to be found in private rented accommodation in Britain, and most likely to be lacking amenities like baths and inside WCs (OPCS 1983). They account for 38 per cent of casual users of DSS Resettlement Units and over 25 per cent of hostel residents in some areas . . . young single Irish people who probably account for a high proportion of those sleeping out in central London (O'Meachair and Burns 1988).
>
> (Harrison and Carr-Hill 1992: 23)

Whoever they are, those Irish people who are represented in the statistics showing high rates of mental illness in the Irish in Britain are not seen as a cause for concern. As Raftery, Jones and Rosato (1990) say:

This evidence has not, however, led to the Irish in Britain being included in current academic discussions of mental illness and ethnicity.

(Raftery, Jones and Rosato 1990: 578)

The generally high mortality rates of Irish people in England cannot be explained in similar fashion to that proposed by Cochrane (1979) for mental illness, however. Raftery Jones and Rosato (1990) draw attention to a complicating factor to be explained in relation to the high SMRs described earlier – the fact that when the Irish in England group is extended to include the English-born children of Irish people they too have a high SMR. This throws doubt on explanations which suggest that the statistics indicating the poor health of Irish people in England are skewed by the presence of a small group of people who are homeless. The inclusion of second-generation Irish makes the size of the Irish population in England about 2.25 million and this group show high SMRs regardless of whether one or both of their parents were born in Ireland. As the RCGP, OPCS and Department of Health study based on consultations (McCormick and Rosenbaum 1990) states:

the 'degree of Irishness' has little effect on the observed raised mortality. Furthermore, this analysis does not support the contention that the overall raised mortality levels in the second generation result solely from social class differences.

(McCormick and Rosenbaum 1990: 120)

The point here is that although some of the raised prevalences in morbidity and raised mortality rates may be explained as being the result of poor health amongst a minority of the Irish in Britain, when the analysis is extended to include the second generation, it becomes unlikely that the overall picture of poor health amongst the Irish in Britain can be attributed to a relatively small group of homeless people. Raftery, Jones and Rosato (1990) again raise the question of whether there may genetic or cultural factors at work which might help to explain the generally poorer health of Irish immigrants and their families.

In order to explore this hypothesis it becomes necessary to study the health of people in Ireland to see whether they too experience higher levels of morbidity and mortality than the English. Reference has already been made to the suggestion by Marmot, Adelstein and Bulusu (1994) that the high rate of deaths from TB in Irish men and women immigrants could be explained by their early experience in Ireland. It therefore becomes necessary to look in more detail at the health of Irish people in Ireland.

Comparison of rates of mental illness at first seemed to suggest that there was something about the Irish or their culture which, even in Ireland, led to a high rate of mental illness. Ni Nuallain, O'Hare and Walsh (1987: 944) summarises the early work by saying:

> For a long time the view has been popular that schizophrenia has been unduly common among the Irish at home (Drapes, 1894; Dawson, 1911) and abroad (Swift, 1913). More recently, psychiatric hospital data showing that first admission rates for schizophrenia were two to three times greater in Ireland than in England and Wales appeared to confirm this view:
>
> (Walsh and Walsh, 1970)

This led to community studies such as as that by Scheper-Hughes (1979) which looked for the explanation in Irish culture. Ni Nuallain, O'Hare and Walsh (1987), however, go on to say that in their study of first admissions the evidence does not support the view that there is a high incidence of schizophrenia in Ireland. A later study by the same authors (Ni Nuallain, O'Hare and Walsh 1990) develops this point and suggests that patients who have recovered from their acute symptoms are, even more often than in other countries, retained in hospital, thus swelling the prevalence rates. This policy of retaining the mentally ill in hospital is changing, though, as in other countries, and more people are now continuing their treatment in the community. The Irish Department of Health Statistics (1990) also show a steady decline in admissions for psychiatric treatment, from 14,000 in 1978 to 9,500 in 1988.

The weight of recent evidence from Irish studies of mental illness in Ireland seems to suggest, then, that the explanation for the raised prevalence of mental illness amongst Irish people in England, which is shown in both hospital- and community-based studies, must be sought in the experience of Irish people in England rather than seeing it simply as part of the risk of being Irish. The essential nature of that experience will be discussed in a later section.

Comparison of the physical health of the Irish in Ireland with that of the Irish in England is also interesting. Overall, life expectancy for both men and women is slightly lower than for England, but not much so (71 years for men as opposed to 71.7, and 76.7 compared to 77.5 for women). The crude death rates, though, which are given for comparative purposes in the Irish Department of Health statistics (1990: 26) are not a very helpful guide in making international comparisons of adult death rates, as the population of Ireland is a very young one with half the population being under 25. World Health Organisation (WHO) figures for 1980–1984 (Statistical Office of European Communities) do suggest, however, that Ireland does have a high SMR compared with the UK and most other European countries. The figures for men being 1,318.7 per 100,000 (UK 1221.8) and for women 850.8 (UK 747.5).

The infant mortality rate has come down in Ireland, as in most other countries, and is comparable with the UK rate (9.2 compared with 9.0, both 1988 figures). The perinatal rate, however, is still high in Ireland.

Comparison of deaths by selected causes does give some grounds for suggesting that the health of people in Ireland, particularly urban dwellers, may be less good than that of people in England. WHO figures indicate that Ireland has a high rate of mortality from tuberculosis, which might help to explain the large number of Irish people in England dying from TB. The figures given are a TB SMR for Ireland of 165 and one of 54 for the UK (1974–1978), but later evidence from Irish Department of Health statistics (1990) shows that deaths from TB are being reduced. The rates have gone down from 7.5 per 100,000 in 1970 to 1.5 in 1990. Cook (1990) notes that the death rate from lung cancer amongst Irish women is the highest in Europe and that the death rate from respiratory diseases for both men and women is the highest in Europe, although it is also high in the UK. In contrast, Irish women had very low rates for cancer of the cervix and the uterus. Cook also draws attention to the fact that men and women in Ireland also had a high death rate from heart disease, the highest in Europe. The UK had the second highest rate though. As well as noting that there is a clear social class gradient in health in Ireland and that there is high rate of unemployment, Cook suggests that the Irish diet is high in animal fat and low in protein, and also notes the increased tendency for urban dwellers in Ireland, both men and women, to be smokers. When the further comparison is made between the health of Irish people in Ireland with that of Irish people in England, it is again clear that although there are differences, for example, the higher rate of mortality from lung cancer and accidents among Irish immigrants to Britain when compared with Irish people in Ireland, when the death rate from all causes is compared, again, there is no clear pattern.

Although the differences in deaths from particular causes are interesting and Cook suggests that there may be differences in diet and lifestyle factors between England and Ireland which may explain these differences in the rates of death from particular causes, there is no definitive evidence to suggest that Irish people in Ireland are much less healthy than English people in England.

The other aspect of health which has to be remembered besides the high mortality rate is the high rate of mental illness of Irish people in England when compared with those of the native English.

We therefore have to return to the problem of how to explain the significantly poorer health of Irish people in England when compared with the native English. As is often the case, no explanation is readily forthcoming from the empirical data but the comparisons which have been made, as well as ruling out some explanations, do suggest some theoretical linkages which are worth exploring.

THEORETICAL EXPLANATION

The theoretical concepts which will be used in this section are those of identity, culture and economic position (class). Although these will be discussed separately, the concepts of identity and culture are quite closely linked. Class is part of a different theoretical perspective but, with culture, it is also one of the factors which shape identity and, through the constraints that low social class places on the opportunities that people have, it also affects their lifestyle.

The history of Ireland and its relationship with England has contributed to the development of a culture and a sense of identity which influences the behaviour and practices of Irish people both in Ireland and in England. That history consists largely of attempts by the English to subjugate the Irish, and Ireland has had for much of the time until 1922 the status of an English colony. Greenslade (1992) draws on the work of Fanon to suggest the effect that this has had on Irish culture and Irish people. Colonised people and their way of life are seen, he suggests, as inferior, and although many of the colonised people are able to resist this view of themselves in their own country, it becomes more difficult when they emigrate. This is particularly so when they emigrate, as many Irish people do, to the country of their colonial oppressors, in this case England. Greenslade uses this argument to explain the high rate of mental illness among the Irish in Britain. A variation of this argument will be used here, but first some aspects of the culture which are more closely related to behaviour will be considered. Although there are signs of change occurring and some (Rossiter 1992) would see the election of Mary Robinson as symbolic of those changes, Irish culture is still based around living in a largely traditional society in which religion plays a significant part in influencing social values, and it may be this which has created the fatalistic attitude in relation to health which McCluskey (1989) has noted. In this study McCluskey, using a health locus of control question, found that as many as 39 per cent of the sample were classified as believing that the state of their health was largely a matter of external control rather than something within their own control. It could be argued that this acceptance of things is related to their experience of being members of the Catholic faith and of living in a traditional, unquestioning society. Similarly, the stoic attitude which made people reluctant to admit to having an illness and pain (Zborowski 1952; Zola 1956; McCluskey 1989), may also be seen as the result of the accepting attitudes developed within Irish culture. Irish people in England showed a similar reluctance to visit a doctor as the RCGP, OPCS, Dept of Health (McCormick and Rosenbaum 1990) study showed. McCluskey (1989) also showed that the majority of the people questioned had a rather traditional and scientifically unsophisticated view of what constituted a healthy diet. Although they thought that good food was an important ingredient of good health, it was not things like a high-fibre diet which were mentioned but fresh food, food which was not canned or processed. This perhaps is a reflection of the fact that many Irish people still have family contacts with the rural agricultural Ireland which has been part of the vision of Ireland which has guided statesmen from the time of de Valera on.

Preserving Ireland as a rural place untainted by the pressures of industrial capitalism has also meant that while some nationalists have seen emigrants as traitors leaving their homeland for selfish reasons, others have given emigrants their blessing and seen emigration as a way of keeping Ireland as a traditional and holy place. This ambivalent attitude towards emigration is something that immigrants have carried with them over the water and it may influence their sense of identity. The experience of the Irish in Ireland has created a culture and a sense of identity which is adapted to that experience but which is less well adapted to the more varied and less traditional pattern of life in England. Ryan (1990) makes the point that

> The average English person tends to have a stage-Irish perception of the migrant, and irrespective of what level of society one entered, from labourer to lecturer, one was likely to be confronted with little jibes ... about the fact one was Irish. Instead of treating this as a bit of fun, many Irish, because of an inferiority complex about England and the English, tended to see it as a continuation of seven hundred years of persecution.
>
> (Ryan, 1990: 55)

He goes on to say that what contributed to their inability to deal with such situations was a 'lack of confidence in their own Irishness' (ibid.).

It is this problem in sustaining or developing their identity in England which will now be used to develop an analysis of how the experience of the Irish in England is central to understanding not just their poor mental health but poor physical health as well.

Irish immigrants to England may come with mixed feelings as a result of the way emigrants have been regarded in Ireland, as indicated previously. Miller (1990) suggests that the out-of-date idea that emigration was a necessary form of exile was encouraged by the middle-class farmers who did not want to share out the land they owned. They were supported by the Catholic Church and the state, who shared a notion that Ireland, a rural country, was a less sinful land than the modern industrial states of England and America, and they thus resisted change. The Church sent them off with blessings and the hope that they would not just retain their faith but also recruit others to Catholicism. The nationalists, however, saw emigration as depopulation and a weakening of the nation. These tensions which have only recently been openly discussed at national level were also reflected at the level of families. Ryan (1990) argues that many immigrants to England came with so many myths and prejudices and the weight of Ireland's experiences with England with them in some form that they arrived with a sense of inferiority towards the English and a lack of faith in their own Irishness.

Whereas in America the Irish were welcomed as fellow republicans who eventually established themselves as Irish-Americans, in England the process of becoming Irish-English has not really been an aim. Irish people in England have tended to keep to their own communities and even there have been slow to organise themselves into anything other than social groupings. Although Jackson (1963: 133) states that 'The institutions of the Irish community in Britain have been perpetuated less from prejudice and the need for mutual protection than they have from sentiment', he accepts that there are ambiguities in these institutions caused by their 'colonial character'. Ryan (1990) believes that the election of Michael O'Halloran to Parliament in 1969 encouraged an increased involvement in national and local politics, but it is still surprising that the Irish in England are not more of a political pressure group in the way that they are in the United States.

What the Irish in England appear to lack as a result of the lack of confidence that Ryan (1990) described is what Antonovsky (1963), following Sartre, calls 'authenticity'. Antonovsky looked at the experience of Jews in America and suggested that:

> The modern emancipated Jew does not know fully who he is, and much of what he does know he cannot accept. He is the stranger who does not wish to be a stranger . . . He retains the old label of Jew but has no identity acceptable to himself. It is this lack of acceptable identity which is the core of the problem for the Jew.
>
> (Antonovsky 1963: 428)

There were times when Jewish people found it possible to be both Jewish and American, when they began to develop a feeling of authenticity, but there were often periods of strain and anxiety. Antonovsky carried out his research into the experience of American Jews at the time the Rosenbergs were charged with and found guilty of espionage. They were sentenced to death by a Jewish-American judge. At such a time Jewish people struggled with their own sense of identity and many wanted to say that the Rosenbergs were communists, not Jews, in order to attempt to preserve their own Jewish-American identity. Similarly, from time to time Irish people in England may be reluctant to be identified as Irish when IRA bombs are exploding in London.

In America the Catholic church and the Irish middle-class did attempt to knit all the Irish immigrants together into communities.

The new culture would adapt some transplanted norms and symbols to both the Irish immigrant experience and the institutions and ideals of middle-class America, creating in the process a new but doubly derivative identity that would transcend the divisions within Irish America.

(Miller 1990: 110)

To what extent these attempts created a sense of authenticity for Irish immigrants and their descendants is not clear, but it does appear that few such attempts were made to create similar Irish organisations in England. Ryan (1990) writing about Irish immigrants to England states that:

Throughout much of this century, there was a complete lack of any organised effort to help the migrant to adjust to life in a new society.

(Ryan 1990: 52)

Danaher (1992) also draws attention to the fact that Catholic schools in England, until 1984, did little to educate their pupils, many of whom were Irish, about their ethnic background and culture.

It seems that many Irish immigrants and their children who were born in England may experience some difficulties in integrating into life in England; they remain, by and large Catholic, even when they intermarry. As Clare Short, the Labour MP says in the book *Working Lives* 'I'm an ethnic Catholic, if you know what I mean' (Holohan 1995: 57). They often return to Ireland for holidays. They never make the physical break from Ireland that the American-Irish do. As Jackson (1963: 159) suggests in a chapter entitled 'Attitudes and anxieties: the problem of prejudice and the problem of identity', 'the proximity of Ireland to the rest of the British Isles [*sic*] ensures that their background retains a strong hold upon them and adds greatly to the difficulties of this marginal citizenship of what has been termed "the Middle Irish Nation"'.

One way of understanding their situation is to suggest that, like Antonovsky's Jews, they experience difficulty in establishing an authentic identity and, as a result, although they mix well as individuals, they have so far failed to identify themselves as a group. They have remained a large number of individuals but have not developed a group identity to give them the sense of security that comes from knowing who you are in an alien land, and which would allow them to take an active part in English life. The 'troubles' in Northern Ireland and bombing activities of the IRA in England made it difficult for Irish people to promote the idea that they are part of a different but legitimate ethnic group with a developing group identity in which individuals could locate themselves. The 'troubles' and the fight for independence have provided the inspiration for many songs and great plays, but the search for identity remains a real one even for people in Ireland. As Tom Paulin writes:

> It has joined the nations of the earth
> but the old people in this baby state
> they whisper Are we fit to govern?
> lookit those swaddlers in their twenties
> they've taken us over
>
> such a struggle to get born – blood in buckets
> bang! wham! the gun and the scaffold
> and then abandoned like this
> left like Oedipus in a handbag
> with no-one to find us or call us worthy

(Paulin 1994: 32)

An article in the *Guardian* draws on a survey carried out by the Action Group for Irish Youth, an English-based group, and suggests that:

> For such young Irish people, questions of identity are clearly not easily resolved. Seeing their residence in Britain as temporary even after seven or eight years, considered permanent emigres back in Ireland, they are viewed by the British as neither foreign nor native.

(Messud 1993: 10)

The Economist (1991) had made a similar point as well as suggesting that even though only a small minority supported the IRA many more felt that they came under suspicion.

What has been suggested in this section is that Irish people coming to England bring with them a traditional culture which includes in it what, following Durkheim, could be seen as collective representations about the English, about Ireland and about the nature of health and illness, all of which influence the way they live and work. This means that although at the level of personal interaction with English people they may experience no sense of hostility, their own interactions with the English are shaped by the collective representations in their culture.

CONCLUSION

From the empirical data it was not possible to single out any one factor which could explain the poorer health of Irish people living in England. The evidence summarised in the first part of this chapter shows that it is unlikely that their poorer health, physical or mental, can be explained by saying that they bring it with them, either as part of their early experience or as part of their genetic make-up. Similarly, whilst it is recognised that first-generation Irish have been overrepresented in the lower social classes, we have insufficient knowledge about the second generation, who also have poor health, to be able to say whether they are also overrepresented in the lower social classes, experiencing the poor housing, for example, that some first-generation people do. The *Labour Force Survey* (Department of Employment 1993) shows that not only do Irish people in England have a higher rate of unemployment than native English, 19 per cent as compared to 12 per cent for men, but that they are also less likely to buy their own house, 56 per cent as compared to 70 per cent of the English. The Labour Force Survey is likely also to understate the poor economic position of the Irish as the survey excludes people living in hostels and institutions, places where many Irish people from nurses to men working in the construction industry may be found.

The poorer economic circumstances and the poor working conditions common to manual workers (40 per cent of London Irish are manual workers) may well contribute to the relatively poor health of Irish people in Britain. These material factors cannot be ignored. Although this class aspect does not seem to be a complete explanation, it is likely that it is a contributory factor in the poor health of Irish people in England. It seems likely that material and cultural factors interact to create a sense of low self-esteem. What can be drawn from the other studies referred to here is the influence of culture. The study of McCluskey (1989) of health beliefs in Ireland, the evidence of the illness behaviour of Irish people in England and their relative reluctance to visit the doctor for non-serious illness suggest a stoic approach which perhaps is not always advisable in the long run. On top of this is the sense of collective insecurity about their identity which may contribute both to their unwillingness to make demands on the health care system and to the likelihood that their problems may eventually emerge as psychological ones, or at least may be diagnosed as such. There is, after all, the possibility that, as has been found to be the case with Afro-Caribbean people, those diagnosing Irish patients may use the stereotypes of Irish people which are commonly found in English culture.

ACKNOWLEDGEMENT

I am grateful to Rory Williams for his comments on an earlier draft of this chapter.

REFERENCES

Adelstein, A., Marmot, M., Dean, G. and Bradshaw, J. (1986a) 'Comparison of mortality of Irish immigrants in England and Wales with that of Irish and British nationals', *Irish Medical Journal* 79(7): 185–189.

Adelstein, A., Marmot, M., Dean, G. and Bradshaw, J. (1986b) 'The Irish in England – do they behave?' Letters to *Irish Medical Journal* 79(11): 331.

Antonovsky, A. (1963) 'Like everyone else, only more so: identity, anxiety and the Jew' in M. Stein, A. Vidich and M. White (eds) *Identity and Anxiety*. USA: Free Press.

Cochrane, R. (1983) *The Social Creation of Mental Illness*. London: Longman.

Cochrane, R. and Bal, S. (1987) 'Migration and schizophrenia: an examination of five hypotheses', *Social Psychiatry* 22: 181–191.

Cochrane, R. and Bal, S. (1989) 'Mental hospital admission rates of immigrants to England: a comparison of 1971 and 1981', *Social Psychiatry* 24: 2–11.

Cochrane, R. and Stopes-Rowe, M. (1979) 'Psychological disturbance in Ireland, in England and in Irish emigrants to England: a comparative study', *Economic and Social Review* 10(4): 301–320.

Cook, G. (1990) 'Health and social inequities in Ireland', *Social Science and Medicine* 31(3): 285–290.

Danaher, N. (1992) 'Irish studies: a historical survey across the diaspora' in P. O'Sullivan (ed.) *The Irish in New Communities, Vol. 2*. London: Leicester University Press.

Department of Employment (1993) *Labour Force Survey*. London: HMSO.

Department of Health (1990) *Health Statistics*. Dublin: Stationery Office.

Economist (1991) 'The Irish in Britain, across the water', 16/3: 28, 31.

Employment Gazette (1994) 'Irish nationals in the British labour market', January: 29–32.

Greenslade, L. (1992) 'White skins, white masks: psychological distress amongst the Irish in Britain' in P. O'Sullivan (ed.) *The Irish in the New Communities, Vol. 2*. Leicester: Leicester University Press.

Harrison, L. and Carr-Hill, R. (1992) *Alcohol and Disadvantage Amongst the Irish in England*. Hull: Department of Social Policy, University of Hull.

Holohan, A. (1995) *Working Lives*. London: The Irish Post.

Jackson, J. (1963) *The Irish in Britain*. London: Routledge & Kegan Paul.

McCluskey, D. (1989) *Health, People's Beliefs and Practices*. Dublin: Stationery Office.

McCormick, A. and Rosenbaum, M. (1990) *Morbidity Statistics from General Practice*. London: HMSO.

Marmot, M., Adelstein, A. and Bulusu L. (1984) *Immigrant Mortality in England and Wales: 1970–1978* (OPCS studies on Population and Medical Subjects No. 47). London: HMSO.

Messud, C. (1993) 'The almost foreign Londoners', *Guardian* 17/3: 10–11.

Miller, K. (1990) 'Emigration, capitalism and ideology in post-famine Ireland' in R. Kearney (ed.) *Migrations: The Irish at Home and Abroad*. Dublin: Wolfhound Press.

Ni Nuallain, M., O'Hare, A. and Walsh, D. (1987) 'Incidence of schizophrenia in Ireland', *Psychological Medicine* 17: 943–948.

Ni Nuallain, M., O'Hare, A. and Walsh, D. (1990) 'The prevalence of schizophrenia in three counties in Ireland', *Acta Psychiatr Scand* 82: 136–140.

OPCS (1990) *Mortality and Geography: A Review in the Mid 1980s* (Series DS No. 9.). London: HMSO.

Owen, D. (1995) *Irish-born People in Great Britain*. Warwick: University of Warwick, Centre for Research in Ethnic Relations.

Paulin, T. (1994) 'Kevin Higgins and the Justice Squad' in T. Paulin *Walking a Line*. London: Faber & Faber.

Raftery, J., Jones, D. and Rosato, M. (1990) 'The mortality of first and second generation Irish immigrants in the U.K.', *Social Science and Medicine* 31(5): 577–584.

Rossiter, A. (1992) 'Between the Devil and the deep blue sea: Irish women, Catholicism and colonialism' in G. Sahgal and N. Yuval-Davis (eds) *Refusing Holy Orders*. London: Virago Press.

Ryan, L. (1990) 'Irish emigration to Britain since World War Two' in R. Kearney (ed.) *Migrations: The Irish at Home and Abroad*. Dublin: Wolfhound Press.

Scheper-Hughes, N. (1979) *Saints, Scholars and Schizophrenics*, Berkeley, CA: University of California Press.

Skrabanek, P. (1986) 'The Irish in England – do they behave?' Letters to *The Irish Medical Journal* 79(11): 331.

Smaje, C. (1995) *Health, 'Race' and Ethnicity*. London: King's Fund Institute.

Walsh, D. and Walsh, B. (1970) 'Mental illness in the Republic of Ireland – first admissions', *Journal of the Irish Medical Association* 63: 365–370.

Willams, R. (1992) 'The health of the Irish in Britain' in W. Ahmad (ed.) *The Politics of Race and Health*. Bradford: Bradford University Race Relations Research Unit.

Zborowski, M. (1952) 'Cultural components in response to pain', *Journal of Social Issues* 8, Fall: 16–30.

Zola, I. (1956) 'Culture and symptoms: an analysis of patients' presenting complaints' in C. Cox and A. Mead (eds) *A Sociology of Medical Practice*. London: Collier-MacMillan.

Chapter 7

Is 'cultural difference' a useful concept?

Perceptions of health and the sources of ill health among Londoners of South Asian origin

Helen Lambert and Leena Sevak

This chapter discusses some research into perceptions of health, ill health and their determinants among people of South Asian origin in London.[1] Qualitative research of this type commonly seeks to investigate and document culturally specific characteristics of particular minority groups, based on an assumption that cultural differences in the UK population that are predictably correlated with ethnic identification significantly affect health status, health-related behaviour and receptivity to health information. In this chapter we question this assumption and suggest that the notion of 'cultural difference' may have limited value in explaining differentials in health status, health beliefs and health-related behaviour in a multi-ethnic society. We argue that this is the result both of reifying, simplistic and unhelpful characterisations of 'culture' which are drawn upon in health and health services research and of narrowly framed methodological approaches to the study of 'ethnic groups', which serve to constrain the nature and interpretation of research findings.

The emphasis placed on behavioural or 'lifestyle' factors to explain the high incidence of chronic conditions has been criticised for 'blaming the victim' while ignoring the socio-economic determinants of ill health (Crawford 1977). This tendency is present in explanations for the causes and approaches to the prevention of particular diseases within the UK population as a whole, but it has been identified as particularly problematic when used to explain the raised prevalence of certain diseases in specific minority ethnic groups (Ahmad 1989, 1992, 1993; Ahmad *et al.* 1989; Pearson 1986: 111–112). In various studies of the health problems of minority ethnic groups, behavioural factors have been implicated while other social determinants such as social class, poverty or racial discrimination have been inadequately controlled for, with the result that the way of life, or 'culture', of the group has been prematurely identified as the 'cause' of the problem (see Ahmad 1993: 19–21) for discussion of this issue as exemplifying the 'racialisation' of health research and Pearson (1986: 102) on the identification of cultural difference with cultural pathology). In the 1980s commentators on the literature on race and health in the UK rightly criticised researchers for having focused on 'exotic' conditions of clinical interest that appeared to be particular to specific minority ethnic groups and were rare in the rest of the population (see, for example, Donovan 1984; Pearson 1986; Philips and Rathwell 1986; Ahmad 1989; Ahmad *et al.* 1989). More recent studies move beyond this narrow approach in so far as they concentrate on conditions (such as hypertension or diabetes) that are responsible for a significant burden of morbidity and mortality and are common in the UK population as a whole. Nevertheless, most health-related social science research among particular minority ethnic groups still arises as a result of epidemiological findings that have demonstrated an increased incidence of these conditions in the groups under study relative to the white population, rather than, for example, as a result of expressed concerns emanating from within these groups (Pearson (1986: 102) and Ahmad (1993: 27) discuss agenda-setting by predominantly white medical professionals).

Our own research evolved out of Leena Sevak's involvement in epidemiological investigations into the high rates of coronary heart disease (CHD) that have been observed among all South Asian migrant groups (McKeigue, Miller and Marmot 1989b; Balarajan 1991). Thus, the work discussed in this chapter stemmed initially from the identification of a particular, biomedically defined health 'problem' that has a high incidence within a specific minority group in the UK. As such, it is characteristic of most social science research in the field of ethnicity and health in that in origin it is epidemiologically driven and policy-related. Unlike epidemiological investigation, however, sociological and anthropological research of this kind is not concerned with identifying and explaining differentials in the distribution of specific diseases. Rather, it is mainly intended to provide relevant information for the planning and provision of appropriate and effective services. The current growth of qualitative research in this area partly reflects an increasing realisation among health professionals that, in an ethnically diverse setting such as the UK, different groups are differentially affected by particular health problems and that people from minority groups may be subject to inappropriate services or to overt or implicit discrimination in gaining access to health services. Particular impetus has been given to such studies by recent shifts in government policy (see Kelleher and Hillier, this volume). While needs assessments of black and minority ethnic groups undertaken by local health authorities usually still consist of biomedically oriented and epidemiologically framed quantitative surveys, awareness of cultural and language specificities has prompted a growing demand for qualitative research that is seen as better able to identify the particular views and attitudes of specific communities than quantitative studies.[2] The demand for service-oriented studies of this nature, though, produces its own difficulties. The first of these is simply that the existence of such studies may be regarded as more important than their findings. The only reason put forward in the *Health of the Nation* White Paper to explain the need for specific studies of minority ethnic groups is that 'information produced for black and ethnic minority groups' needs to be 'culturally and linguistically sensitive' (Department of Health 1993: 121). Conceivably, the act of commissioning research into perceptions of health and health services among specific groups may itself be used as a means to demonstrate that sufficient attention is being given to these 'sensitivities', while the results of the research are largely disregarded in policy design (Philips and Rathwell 1986: 17) or are utilised selectively to support prior decisions about resource allocation (cf., Stubbs 1993: 47). Other problems engendered by a growing demand for qualitative health research focused on particular minority ethnic groups include the ways that research findings themselves may be shaped by the initial framing of the research agenda to ensure 'policy relevance' and by prior assumptions about cultural difference. We illustrate these problems by presenting work derived from two interlinked studies into perceptions of coronary heart disease and diabetes among several groups of South Asian origin in London, followed by a critical discussion of this material. To provide some background information, we start with a brief review of some general character-istics of the relevant South Asian communities in London, before turning to a description of the methodological approaches adopted in the research.

STUDY COMMUNITIES

In the course of the two studies three geographical areas were chosen so as to sample each of the three communities under study: Camden (Bangladeshi), Wembley (Gujarati) and Southall (Punjabi). The average socio-economic status of these three groups is highest in Gujaratis, intermediate in Punjabis and lowest in Bangladeshis. Most Gujarati migrants arrived from East Africa in the 1960s and 1970s; smaller numbers migrated directly from the state of Gujarat in western India. Gujaratis are predominantly Hindu with a smaller number of Muslims. Gujaratis living in North-west London are mostly well-educated, with a high proportion of self-employed businessmen, managers and professionals compared to other South Asian groups. The main language spoken is Gujarati with Kutchi Gujarati spoken by Ismailis.

Punjabis settled in Southall in two waves also: first, from the northern Indian state of Punjab in the 1950s, then from East Africa in the 1960s and 1970s. Both men and women work mainly in skilled manual jobs around Southall, with a smaller proportion in family businesses such as retail and catering. About 75 per cent of Punjabis living in Southall are Sikhs, with smaller numbers of Hindus and Muslims. Muslims in Southall originate mainly from the Punjab province of Pakistan and from northern India. Colloquial Urdu/Hindi is a 'link language' across most of northern India and Pakistan, and almost all first-generation migrants from Gujarat, Punjab and Kashmir speak this as a second language.

Bangladeshi Muslims are the most homogeneous of the three communities, mostly originating from rural areas in the province of Sylhet in northern Bangladesh. The first migrants from Bangladesh were unaccompanied men, who arrived during the late 1950s and settled in what is now the London borough of Tower Hamlets. From the early 1970s these men were joined by their wives and children in increasing numbers. The demographic make-up of first-generation Bangladeshi migrants in the UK is unusual, with a marked age difference between husbands and wives and a high proportion of unaccompanied men in middle age. Many had worked as cooks in the merchant shipping fleet, and the main sources of employment for this group are the catering and clothing industries. Bangladeshi migrants are more socio-economically deprived than other migrant groups. Levels of literacy among first-generation migrants are low. Bangladeshis are isolated not only from the native British population but also from other groups of South Asian origin. One reason for this is that Urdu/Hindi is not a second language for most Bangladeshi migrants, who speak the Sylheti dialect of Bengali and sometimes standard Bengali.

BACKGROUND TO THE STUDIES

The studies from which our material is derived were carried out at different time periods and funded by two separate agencies with particular views of the purpose and use of information obtained from such research. We include details of the methods and funding sources of both studies for two reasons; first, as a means of illustrating the significance of methodological differences in research design on research findings, and second, in order to ground our observations in a broader comparative framework than that provided by analysis of a single study. The first piece of research followed the completion of a large cohort study investigating the aetiology of CHD among South Asian and European men in which Leena Sevak was involved as a nutritionist. The results of this epidemiological research suggested weight loss and increased physical activity as possible interventions for prevention of CHD. The qualitative research was planned in order to study existing perceptions of causes and prevention of heart disease in the community so that such interventions could be appropriately formulated. At this time the Department of Health was prepared to support research to produce and pre-test health education material on prevention of CHD for South Asian communities. As the South Asian community in Britain is heterogeneous, two sub-groups – Gujarati and Punjabi – were included in the original grant proposal to the Department of Health. The selection of these two sub-groups was largely determined by the languages spoken by the researcher and by time constraints. The main aims were to explore the feasibility of conducting such a study in South Asian communities in London using qualitative methods and to investigate diversity in views on health between these two South Asian sub-groups.

Funding was agreed on condition that Bangladeshis were also included in the sampling frame. The reason put forward by the funding body for doing so was that Bangladeshis were particularly deprived and had worse health than other South Asian groups. This argument appeared to be based on the view that the study should not be seen to exclude this particular community, rather than on considerations of the feasibility of conducting such a study in the short time period for which funding was offered (six months) or the quality of the information that would be obtained. The study was carried out between November 1991 and April 1992 and, in accordance with funding criteria, attempted to test health education materials about coronary heart disease among groups of first-generation Bangladeshi, Punjabi and Gujarati men and women.

Because of its specific aims, this study had a relatively narrow focus and the same questions were put to all participants in a well-structured format. During the course of the analysis, it became clear that a broader knowledge of sociocultural context was necessary in order fully to understand concepts and responses to health and disease. Some further research on related issues using a different methodological approach was developed in collaboration with Helen Lambert, who had conducted anthropological research on lay perceptions and practices relating to health both in North India and among white British people in England. One research project in Southall is continuing and the results of that study are not discussed in this chapter. The second study, which we consider here, investigated a broader range of issues relating to ideas about the causes and prevention of CHD exclusively among Gujaratis living in Brent and was commissioned by Central and North West London Health Promotion Unit. Their specific concern was to acquire information that would have direct relevance for the formulation and modification of CHD-prevention strategies among Gujaratis in Brent. This study was also funded for six months and was carried out between November 1993 and April 1994.

RECRUITMENT AND METHODS OF DATA COLLECTION

In both studies it was decided to contact and interview participants in non-health related settings to avoid bias in responses arising from an institutional environment. In the first study one general practice in Southall (Punjabi) and three in Wembley (Gujarati) were used to make initial contact with potential participants from these groups as they waited to consult their doctors. The selection criteria were that interviewees should be adults between the ages of 35 and 64 without previous history of heart disease. Recruiting participants from Bangladeshi communities proved to be more difficult. After consulting with Bangladeshi community groups, it was decided not

Table 7.1 Socio-demographic characteristics of the participants (n = 32)

| | Bangladeshi | | Gujarati | | Punjabi | |
	Men	Women	Men	Women	Men	Women
Age						
35–44	—	1	2	4	3	5
45–65	4	2	4	2	3	2
Total	4	3	6	6	6	7
Education						
school level	4	2	1	3	3	4
higher	—	—	5	3	3	3
none	—	1	—	—	—	—
Employment						
employed	3	—	6	3	6	5
unemployed	1	—	—	1	—	—
housewife	—	3	—	2	—	2
Housing						
owner occupier	—	—	5	5	6	6
council rented	4	3	—	—	—	1
private rented	—	—	1	1	—	—
Languages						
mother tongue only	2	3	—	1	2	6
mother tongue plus English	2	—	6	5	4	1

to use general practices but to identify potential participants by using the random walk method in the London Borough of Camden. Although time-consuming, this method proved more successful than first establishing contact at general practices and arranging a subsequent interview in the participant's home.

In this first study a short questionnaire was completed at the first meeting to collect information about the participant's age, occupation, languages spoken, education level attained, whether suffering from diabetes or heart disease and whether and where they had come across any health education information regarding prevention of heart disease. Table 7.1 gives some details of the study sample. From the men and women contacted, four separate focus groups were convened, comprising between four and eight participants, in

Southall and Wembley. All meetings took place at a local community centre, and as far as possible meetings were organised at weekends during the daytime. In all three communities focus groups had to be organised twice because of poor attendance. The main reasons given for non-attendance were shift work and lack of time. Discussion meetings were convened twice with Bangladeshi participants, but we were not successful in obtaining adequate attendance rates. All the focus groups were convened before in-depth interviews were conducted. Interviews were carried out using a questionnaire schedule developed from the experience with focus groups.

The individual interviews with Bangladeshi men and women were conducted with the help of a Sylheti-speaking interpreter and all other interviews were conducted by LS in Gujarati or Punjabi, as appropriate. Interviews were conducted in the informants' homes (as far as possible, alone with the informant) and took between 40 minutes and one and a half hours. All interviews and discussions were taped, transcribed and translated into English. Participants were interviewed about their beliefs concerning health in general and heart disease in particular, with a focus on issues such as prevention, causes and personal attributes of those affected by heart disease and diabetes. The interviews were introduced as being largely about health and utilised a questionnaire schedule but allowed open-ended responses so as to obtain discursive material regarding health as a value, control over health, appropriate response to ill health, the possible prevention of illness, actual experiences of ill health both of the subject and of their family and friends, obesity and physical exercise.

Very little currently available health promotion material from the Look After Your Heart Campaign and other programmes intended to reduce the risk of coronary heart disease has been specifically designed for use in South Asian communities. The main product specifically for South Asian communities was the Health Education Authority's video tape 'Action on coronary heart disease in Asians', available in English, Hindi/Urdu and Bengali. This video was shown at the end of each focus group meeting and also at the end of each interview, usually in the company of other members of the household. The video session was followed by a further discussion, to which other household members contributed. By using a video tape rather than written health education material, it was possible to study the responses of informants without the complications which arise from literacy problems, which are especially common among older women.

A more flexible approach was taken in the second study in order to gain a broader understanding of the lives of the study participants. Investigative methods included semi-structured interviews, informal group discussions and a limited amount of participant observation in local community centres. Initial contact with potential interviewees was made both at general practices, while they waited to consult their doctors, and at community organisations. Three general practices and three community organisations based in the north and south of Brent were used, and those who agreed to participate were given a letter explaining the purpose of the study. A distribution of participants across the whole borough was considered to be important since south Brent is generally more economically deprived than the northern part of the borough. The names and addresses of potential interviewees were taken and an appointment for interview was made later by telephone. All except one interview took place in the individual's home. A total of 55 informants initially agreed to participate in the study, of which seven informants were excluded as they were not Gujaratis; all the contacts made at one health centre had to be excluded as all those who agreed were Punjabi Muslims. Of the 48 eligible informants who initially gave consent to be included in the study, 29 agreed to be interviewed on subsequent contact. Lack of time and other commitments were the main reasons given for declining to participate in the study. Seven of those interviewed were contacted through local community organisations and 22 through their general practice. Two of the interviews were with carers whose wives were disabled and in both cases discussion inevitably centred on the immediate concerns of these individuals, so that little information of direct relevance to the study was obtained. Opportunistic unstructured discussions at local community groups were also used to explore issues related to general health. Participant observation took place at regular open days held at a local Asian women's centre and in a community group providing reflexology treatment sessions. These were not recorded, but notes were made immediately following these sessions. All individual interviews and group discussions were conducted in either Gujarati or English, depending on the preference of the participants. Those with higher education or currently studying preferred to speak in English, but the majority of the participants preferred to speak in Gujarati. On average, interviews took between

Table 7.2 Socio-economic characteristics of Gujarati participants (n = 29)

	Age		Education			Employment			
	19–80	17–72	school	higher	none	employed	unemployed	housewife	student
Men	12	—	6	5	1	6	5	—	1
Women	—	17	10	5	2	8	4	3	2
Total	12	17	16	10	3	14	9	3	3

40 minutes and one hour and all were recorded, transcribed and translated into English. The interviews were semi-structured, using a checklist of questions and topics to ensure that areas of interest were covered, including discussion of specific topics such as knowledge of risk factors, control over risk factors, perceived barriers to risk reduction and knowledge of existing sources of health information. Perceptions of body shape and body image were also explored by showing a series of line drawings of male and female figures with varying weight-for-height and waist-to-hip ratios. Table 7.2 gives details of some characteristics of the individual interviewees in the second study. The ages of interviewees ranged from 17 to 80 years. All the participants were Gujarati Hindus from different castes. Although there are other Gujarati religious groups living in Brent, none were encountered during the study period. This may be because they organise separately and/or use different general practices from those selected for recruitment of participants; most of the Muslims at two of the local health centres used Muslim GPs whereas Hindus predominantly attended surgeries run by Hindu GPs. Of the male interviewees, all except two lived in the north of the borough. Most were married with children and owned their homes; all except two lived in nuclear families and some had members of their extended family living in the area. All the men but one were first-generation immigrants from East Africa or India. All of the women interviewees who lived in north Brent were home owners or lived with their parents, whereas all of those who lived in south Brent were council tenants except for one, who was homeless and living in temporary accommodation. All those who worked were employed in unskilled manual jobs and worked shifts. All the women except one were literate in Gujarati.

In the first study the method that was employed limited possible reponses to the questions asked. In the second study, although a checklist of questions pertaining to particular topics was used, informants were also encouraged to talk about their everyday experiences of work, relationships, support networks, use of home remedies and sources of information. This approach made it possible to gain a better understanding of the constraints placed upon individuals due to their particular social and economic circumstances and the ways in which life experiences may shape views of health maintainance and disease prevention. In addition, the use of informal group discussions and participant observation gave an opportunity to verify information obtained during individual interviews.

Although the approach used in the second study in Brent generated more contextualised information which helped to build a picture of the study participants' lives, the results of the two studies were none the less broadly similar in terms of perceptions of causes and prevention of illness in general and heart disease in particular. Moreover, although the data were collected using different methods in a total of three different sub-groups of South Asian origin, our overall results showed little difference between the sub-groups regarding these perceptions. Accordingly, the data are discussed as a whole with specific reference made to the source only where significant differences were present between the studies, either in the way material was elicited or in the responses given by members of particular sub-groups.

FINDINGS

In our discussion of the findings from these two studies, we begin with a summary of data concerning CHD but go on to focus in more detail on some more general material concerning concepts of health, its maintenance and the causes of disease among lay people of South Asian origin from a variety of backgrounds. Although this choice results partially from the fact that some of our more specific findings pertaining to coronary heart disease have been presented elsewhere (Sevak and Lambert 1994; Sevak and McKeigue 1993; McKeigue and Sevak 1994), it is also intended as a corrective to predominant approaches in the study of ethnicity and health as described above. Since much qualitative research in this field is contract-based and policy-driven, it tends to focus on knowledge, perceptions and practices relating to a particular disease or 'health problem'. For lay people, however, ideas pertaining to a particular disease may be shaped by general health-related concepts and experiences as much as by 'disease-specific' knowledge.

Causes of heart disease

In the first study questions regarding causes of heart disease were asked directly in order to elucidate knowledge of risk factors. In the second study most informants mentioned their concern about heart disease without any prompting. Almost all the participants were aware of heart disease as a major health problem among South Asian people. Heart disease was mostly spoken of in relation to a known individual who had suffered from the disease. Like other illness, heart disease was considered to be caused by interactions between several factors, the most frequently mentioned of which was mental stress. The main sources of mental stress were identified as financial difficulties and interpersonal relationships. The other major factors mentioned were smoking, dietary fat, alcohol intake and hard physical labour. From the range of responses in both studies it was clear there was a general familiarity with health education information regarding the causes of heart disease. However, although risk factors for heart disease were listed 'correctly', informants expressed scepticism about their relevance to their own lives when knowledge of medical risk factors derived from health education information was directly compared with personal knowledge of actual cases of heart disease. The lifestyles of known individuals who had heart disease were compared and contrasted with medically defined 'risk factors' and doubts about health education messages concerning the prevention of heart disease were expressed where a 'fit' with these medical risk factors in actual cases was not apparent. Known individuals who had suffered the sudden onset of heart disease in the absence of medically defined risk factors were cited to illustrate the fact that the occurrence of heart disease did not conform to health professionals' explanations of risk. For example, a Gujarati man disputed that there were particular sorts of people who were more at risk than others on these grounds:

> Even youngsters of 26 years get it. I had someone like that who worked with me. Heart attack has nothing to do with fatness, age. It can happen anytime, whether you are fat or thin or young or old it does not matter.

In addition, health education messages were seen as constantly changing and this was often given as a reason for not believing them. A Gujarati woman stated the causes of heart disease as follows:

Heart disease is caused by drinking and smoking and cholesterol. Cholesterol from fat like ghee, oil and fried foods. But they say all sorts of things but I don't believe it all. Because they keep changing their minds.

The nature of health

Informants were asked if they considered themselves healthy and how they defined health. Most informants considered themselves to be healthy if they did not experience any symptoms and defined health in terms of function, placing emphasis on body movement, ability to perform everyday functions without pain or difficulty, absence of 'illness', as illustrated in the following statement by a Punjabi woman:

Health means you haven't got any illness. You are healthy and perfect. If you have got disease or other things, if you have got a headache and your stomach aches, your leg hurts you are not healthy.

Although health was generally defined as functional capacity and absence of illness, respondents expressed considerable uncertainty about the underlying state of the body, and being healthy was at least partly attributed to luck or chance. A Gujarati man explained:

Health is: we are working, we are fit, we can walk. But you can't say when something happens. So you can't say, we can say that we are healthy because we are not taking any tablets but anything can happen any time . . . no one knows.

To explore beliefs about influences on health in general, informants were asked 'What things in people's lives are bad for their health?' The same question was then asked specifically in relation to informants' own lives. The focus on this issue in the research derived both from the fact that intervention strategies for the prevention of coronary heart disease mainly focus on the notion of individual behavioural change and from a critical awareness that South Asians in general – and Hindus in particular – have, in common with the working class (Pill and Stott 1987), often been represented as 'fatalistic'. Given funders' expectations and the influential place of psychological theories such as the Health Belief Model (Rosenstock 1974; Janz and Becker 1984) in health professionals' views of lay knowledge and practices, it was necessary to address these assumptions directly in our research. However, it is important to note that the focus on 'individual control over/responsibility for health' is primarily a product of these research imperatives rather than a finding that emerged naturally from informants' unprompted concerns. By contrast, responses to a general question about possible causes of ill health produced unprompted reference to a wide range of influences.

Sources of ill health

Asked, 'What do you think causes ill health?', the influences that our informants cited ranged from the social situation of the individual and economic pressures to environmental pollution, stress and diet. These influences, then, include both 'external' causes over which individuals can have little or no control and 'internal' ones that may be open to individual modification. Our informants made no explicit distinction between these two types of cause, but in their responses exposure to such 'external factors' in the UK was often emphasised as a contrast with life in the country of origin. A Gujarati man's description was typical of the responses which attributed ill health to the effects of aspects of the environment in Britain:

> Well in this country we don't get what we need, firstly we don't have fresh food, we don't get fresh vegetable, fresh air. In the house there is double glazing on the window and doors and we sit inside and no one wants to open it, so we breathe in air that is not good for our health.

The next three sections examine in further detail the constituents of health and causes of ill health that were most emphasised by informants.

Eating patterns

A great deal of emphasis was placed by most informants upon eating 'healthy foods' such as fresh vegetables, fruits and pulses in order to maintain general health. The importance of a regular lifestyle was often voiced and inappropriate timing of meals was regarded as especially important in contributing to illness generally. The meal pattern in Britain was compared with that in India and East Africa where the main meal of the day is consumed at noon.

A female informant explained the importance of changes in meal times:

> [Here we] eat at night. After meals we just go to bed. No one does any kind of exercise after the meals. Therefore everything is jammed. In Kenya we used to eat in the afternoon, by the night you have digested it, had some kind of exercise and work.

Informants in all of the sub-groups also considered the South Asian diet to be particularly high in fat and several informants believed (incorrectly) that fat intake among South Asians was higher than in Europeans. A Punjabi woman explained:

> We eat a lot of fried food. White people don't eat that much. They only eat fish and chips which are fried. But we people follow them and eat fish and chips and also parathas [fried chapatis]. In our sabzi [vegetables] and meat we put too much ghee. It has less water but more ghee or oil.

Climate and physical activity

The effect of climate on health and contrasts between the UK climate and that of the country of origin were also mentioned by most informants. The effect of heat from the sun was regarded as beneficial for health, especially in facilitating the digestive process. A hot climate was also said to melt body fat and cleanse the body of poisons through the action of sweating. In addition, an emphasis was placed on the greater degree of physical exercise involved in work within the country of origin in comparison with that in Britain. Both of these factors were both seen as affecting proper digestive function and were put forward to explain resulting weight gain and health problems in Britain. A Gujarati woman explained the drawbacks of the English climate and limited exercise in comparison to that of India:

> Because we do not get the sun over here, our body cannot digest [food] and causes health problems. Here due to lack of sun you cannot digest, you do not exercise. In India you work all day, you sweat and feel much lighter. All the rubbish is thrown out in heat and sweat. It stays in your body as in a freezer in this country.

Similarly, another female informant observed:

> In this country due to cold weather we cannot digest [food]. In

Kenya due to the heat and work we could digest, here we cannot digest it and we also eat at night.

Psycho-social stress

Almost all informants cited what they variously called 'worry', 'tension', 'pressure' or 'stress' as responsible for ill health. The English words were often used even by those who did not speak much English. The following quote from a Punjabi woman is typical of such views:

> More than anything else, it is worry, whether it is a man or woman . . . worry is the cause of so many diseases. If you have no worries, you are healthy. This is the root cause of all illnesses.

While no explanations were offered as to the mechanisms through which worry may produce bodily ill health, respondents characteristically assumed the non-separability of mind and body and referred to interaction and mutual influences between them in statements such as, 'stress changes people's behaviour', and, '[stress] makes all the functions of the body weak'. Worry and tension were ascribed to a variety of factors, including financial burdens, unemployment, poor housing, social isolation, conflict with children and racial discrimination. Financial difficulties were most often cited as causing mental stress, as a Gujarati man who had been made redundant explained:

> There are two reasons for this, the living standard is high and there is less income. So mental pressure increases. At present this is government policy. It is very difficult. Can you pay the mortgage? How can a husband and wife live on £90? Can you heat your house in winter? If you are unemployed what can you do?

Some informants spoke of responsibility for their extended families in India. This was cited as a cause of added financial difficulties as well as a source of conflict among those who were providing the support from here. Stress was also ascribed to long working hours and the pace of life in Britain, as a Gujarati informant reported:

> What happens is that, we said everyone is in tension. The reason is that we are going to work in the morning, some go at 6 a.m. some at 7. Some go far, rushing all the time, and some come late and worry about missing their bus and being late for work. All

day they are in tension that, will I be able to get to work? And
then you come home and you are tired. You don't even have time
to sit and talk to your family. And if anyone says anything you
feel why did they say that to me because you are under tension so
I am talking about this country, so no one has time to sit and
relax. When it is Saturday then you have to go shopping and you
run around.

Although racial discrimination was regarded as a source of problems in acquiring housing and employment, it was not a prominent
topic of discussion and was rarely connected directly with health
problems. Given that the interviewer was herself of South Asian
origin, the assumption of shared experiences may have led to an
underplaying of this aspect of life in London. Another plausible
explanation is that individuals give more weight to sources of stress
affecting health which are experienced on an everyday basis, such
as financial responsibilities or family problems, than to those, such
as incidences of racism, which are experienced only sporadically
(especially in areas such as Brent and Southall where a substantial
proportion of the population are of South Asian origin). Racism
can be a structural cause of stressors such as financial worries due
to discrimination in employment recruitment, but is not perceived
as bearing so directly on individual health as resulting forms of
economic disadvantage.

Informants of both sexes frequently attributed ill health to worry
and tension. However, women's perceived stress was never directly
related to themselves but always to the situation of the rest of the
family, as illustrated by statements such as: 'I think it is all to do
with the family' or 'If everybody is happy then automatically your
health is well'. Indeed, in general when talking about the importance of health, women related it to the family and considered the
impact of illness on the whole family. Men, by contrast, generally
expressed concern about their health in relation to personal illness.
They tended to emphasise their conditions of employment and the
effect of 'hard work' or 'hard labour' on health, either as physically
demanding or as mentally taxing work involving responsibility for
others. Informants recalled the difficulties they had faced as new
immigrants, such as discrimination in access to housing. These
difficulties were seen as having taken a toll on health. In the words
of a Punjabi man:

Also people of our age group – we were pioneers. We came here in the beginning in this country and we had nothing, the majority did not have anything. I came with £5. I had £5 exchange money. Worked day and night. We had housing problems, sometimes did not get rented rooms. All this, we have achieved all this through hard work.

Bangladeshi men were the only group who identified socio-economic deprivation as an adverse influence on their own health. They also emphasised the effects of anxiety and tension resulting from economic difficulties. Since Bangladeshis experience more socio-economic deprivation than any other group, it is not surprising that these perceptions are common.

Control over and responsibility for health

In spite of the emphasis placed on various forms of environmental and structural determinants of health status, most informants also expressed the view that people could to some extent affect their own state of health. Regulating food, lifestyle, exercise, smoking and alcohol consumption were seen as the most important means of maintaining health. Control over these factors was mainly seen as being achieved through will-power. A Gujarati woman explained how one can influence one's own health:

If the person makes up his mind that I want to improve my health and not eating this food is good for me [because] doctor says so, friends say so. So if we control our minds we can do that – why not?

Even those who regarded health as primarily a matter of fate, chance or divine will qualified these opinions by expressing a belief in the individual ability to influence health status and the import-ance of information and 'doctor's advice'. In the words of a Gujarati man:

Some people will say it is in the hands of God. But having said that there is some contribution from oneself to how you live. There is not absolute control, if man had control over disease then nobody can die.

Similarly, a Bangladeshi woman in the study attributed illness to God, but at the same time stated the importance of individual action:

> Illness depends on Allah, but one can take care of it. If I do not care about it, maybe it will increase very badly. Say I have fallen ill, some disease has attacked me, if I do not try to control over it, it will advance in its own way. Always have courage in mind, never be afraid of the illness.

To ascertain whether and under what circumstances an individual might be held responsible for becoming ill, in interviews informants were asked, 'If someone gets ill, is it ever their own fault? How?' Most informants stated that sometimes, under specific circumstances, an individual can be held responsible for their ill health, but responses to the question suggested a complex understanding of individual responsibility for health. Individuals whose actions were considered to be harmful to their health were blamed for their illness, with smoking, drinking alcohol and generally being careless most often being cited as 'bad habits'. On the other hand, cases of illness that were unattributable to personal living habits were also repeatedly cited to exemplify a broader principle that individuals cannot generally be held responsible for becoming ill.

Here, too, gender differences were apparent: women tended to consider themselves responsible not only for their own health but that of their household as well, and viewed illness as having a detrimental impact on the family as a whole. Men, by contrast, tended to speak of illness in personal terms. Some Punjabi Sikh informants referred to the body as a temple to God which should not be abused or damaged. This philosophy is regarded as the basis for the prohibition of smoking in Sikhism. A Punjabi man explained:

> God has given us this body, so to keep it healthy is our responsibility. It is like a house – a building. If you put good material into this house it will be good strong house. The kind of food you eat will accordingly give you a body and health. This is your responsibility.

While this view may be specific to a particular religious faith, in the understanding of health maintenance as a combination of divine providence and personal responsibility it is similar to the views of other Muslim and Hindu informants cited above.

Constitution and heredity

The notion of constitutional predisposition as influential in determining whether individuals become ill was mentioned by informants in all three communities. This included both a recognition of genetic inheritance among kin as an influential cause of particular health problems and a more subtle view of individually specific inherent predisposition. The latter was described in phrases such as 'natural tolerance in your body', 'it is from your birth' or 'child is born with a weakness', or occasionally by the word *tasir* (constitution). The quote below from a Gujarati man links heredity, expressed by reference to blood, with susceptibility to mental ill health:

> And also everyone's blood is different, so it is said. Sometimes the blood is such from the beginning that you get affected by depression more, and your partner's blood may be different and they don't get affected . . . groups are different.

Although heredity was regarded as important, environmental factors were perceived as interacting with hereditary susceptibility to disease. A Gujarati man explained:

> Blood pressure is like this, it is inherited. Father has it, forefathers had it so you are going to get blood pressure and also . . . people have to pay mortgage and bills, so they have that sort of tension so blood pressure goes high.

Apart from the notion of heredity, the inherent nature of one's constitution (*prakruti* or *tasir* in Gujarati in the Brent study) was also cited as an attribute which made some people more susceptible to certain diseases than others or which, conversely, determined individual resistance to adverse circumstances in general. One Punjabi informant reported that:

> To my knowledge, see, there are various kinds of people. There are some who do not feel anything, no worries, no temper. Whilst others can't tolerate anything at all. See there are 50–55, some can some can't.

More specifically, constitution was cited as explaining individual differences in physical capacity to resist and to recover from illness. A 21-year-old woman stated:

> Yes I think it depends on the constitution and some people do have weak constitutions than others. A constitution is your, I suppose your ability, your resilience, how resilient you are, your inner strength. Some people recover very fast than others.

The idea of differences in body constitution was sometimes expressed by reference to the Gujarati proverb, '*tunde tunde mati judi*', (every head has different intelligence), or was discussed in terms of the tri-humoral theory of classical Indian medicine as the inherent tendency for a particular humoral imbalance. A Gujarati woman explained:

> If something you cannot digest, like some people can't digest some things. They get *pitta* [humoral 'phlegm'], such as some people can't digest cucumber if they eat at night and some people can eat it because everybody's *tasir* [constitution] is different.

Some informants also expressed the opinion that Indian people have a different constitution from the native British and, since they are not sufficiently acclimatised, should take particular care of what they eat. Such views are linked with the notions of environmental and climatic influence referred to above, as illustrated by a Gujarati woman's explanation:

> In frozen [food] they add some chemicals, I don't know what it is called, but they affect our health. These English people, they are born and brought up over here and have been living on it for ages therefore it doesn't affect them that much. Why, because they are snow people, we are from hot climate, we have hot blood, so this food does not suit us.

Perceptions of medical treatment

Although views of the health services were not the main focus of these studies, a substantial body of data on this topic was collected during the course of our research. This cannot be discussed in any detail in this chapter, but the interlinking of bodily health, environmental influence and 'lifestyle' in informants' views is well illustrated by their comments about medical treatment. A frequent complaint about treatment was lack of advice about food when medicines were prescribed. Dietary modification is an integral part of treatment in both traditional Ayurvedic medicine and in popular responses to ill health in South Asia, and among our informants too there was an expectation that doctors should give advice about appropriate diet when prescribing medicine. A Gujarati man related his experience of his GP as follows:

See, if he properly checks up everything and accordingly gives you the appropriate medicine, then there is no problem. These doctors after giving you the medicine will never tell you or guide you about food and its effects, what to eat and not to eat. They are only concerned about how many patients they have to see and how to finish all that and end it.

DEGREES OF DIFFERENCE IN HEALTH-RELATED CONCEPTS AND THEIR RELEVANCE TO HEALTH POLICY AND PLANNING

Our discussion of these research findings first compares and contrasts various groups in order to examine the differences that may exist between them. The vexed issue of cultural homogeneity is a legitimate concern of both funders and researchers and has particular significance for research among people of South Asian origin. Health professionals are now generally cognisant of the fact that ethnic minorities do not constitute monolithic entities and that among people of South Asian origin there are major differences of religion, language and culture (McKenzie and Crowcroft 1994; Senior and Bhopal 1994). This, indeed, is one reason that the studies discussed in this chapter received funding from institutions in the health sector. None the less, recognition of heterogeneity is in practice constrained by policy considerations. The utility of studies carried out in order to provide local health services with information about perceived needs or attitudes to particular diseases is directly related to their translatability into practical recommendations for the provision of appropriate information and services. While health providers become increasingly aware of 'cultural difference', resource limitations constrain the degree to which heterogeneity can be acknowledged in practice.[3] On the other hand, given the dearth of systematic comparative studies and the methodological difficulties in undertaking such research, this presumed heterogeneity is largely putative. While language, dietary and religious distinctions and even variations in the prevalence and incidence of particular health problems between different groups sharing South Asian origins can be readily observed, whether these significantly affect (for instance) views of disease prevention or the use of health services is largely unknown. Both health status and attitudes towards prevention are known to be correlated with economic status (Townsend and Davidson 1982; Rocheron, Dickinson and Kahn

1989) and racial discrimination can certainly affect attitudes to and use of health services (Bowler 1993). The general assumption among health professionals has however been that *cultural* differences within the UK population significantly affect health status, health-related behaviour and receptivity to health information. This assumption is a 'common-sense' one among health professionals, for whom cultural difference constitutes deviance from the cultural norms of the dominant group and so is readily equated with pathology (Khan 1979; Goel *et al.* 1981), but it is poorly verified. Yet the very purpose of research into the cultural aspects of health within particular groups produces an inherent bias in the interpretation of research findings. Regardless of whether they are initiated by health authorities or by social researchers, funding for studies of health-related perceptions (attitudes, beliefs, ideas) is usually obtained on the grounds that the research will produce findings to facilitate the provision of more appropriate, acceptable and therefore effective health service delivery, health education materials or health promotion strategies for the group under investigation. This creates a tendency for findings to be interpreted by reference to supposed culturally specific beliefs and practices, particularly when comparative investigation of other local groups is not part of the study.

The issue of 'cultural difference' can, however, be regarded as an empirical question, although how differences between groups are conceptualised obviously depends on the definition of such 'groups' and on the selection of groups for comparison. Comparative analysis of our research findings focuses on three sets of salient contrasts: between sub-groups of South Asian origin; between South Asians in the UK and those in the region of origin; and between South Asians in the UK and the indigenous white population.[4] This analysis raises queries about the relative significance of cultural differences in understanding health-related perceptions and formulating strategies for health promotion and disease prevention.

At the first level is the question of whether there are cultural differences between groups of people of South Asian origin that significantly influence health-related ideas and behaviour. The findings from our second study concerning knowledge of risk factors and concepts relating to prevention of heart disease among Hindu Gujaratis in Brent were very similar to the findings of the first study that focused on selected Punjabi, Bangladeshi and Gujarati communities in London, as were most general ideas pertaining to disease prevention and the causes of ill health. The most distinctive difference was between Sylhetis and the other groups studied, in that Sylhetis placed greater emphasis on housing as their primary concern and expressed relative lack of interest in disease prevention generally. This finding can most plausibly be attributed to the poor living conditions among this group who are, significantly, the most recently arrived migrants. However, this groups are also Muslims and the relative lack of concern that informants from this group expressed for health issues overall, suggests some similarities with others in the study who also expressed disinterest in discussing prevention on the grounds that one's health is 'in God's hands'. A few of our Gujarati Hindu and Sikh women informants expressed similar views in relation to the prevention of disease and this might suggest that religiosity in general rather than adherence to a particular religious faith is the source of these views (cf. Donovan 1986: 123 who reports similar findings for her religious informants). The possibility that the distinctive concerns found to be present among Sylhetis are related to their religious faith rather than to their status as recent immigrants living in poverty, however, would require further research, and even a finding that other Muslim groups of differing economic status express similar ideas would not in itself demonstrate that this is a characteristically Muslim view. Moreover, to interpret their statements about the relative unimportance of individual preventive action as 'fatalism' (Donovan 1986: 123) would be incorrect. As illustrated in the quotations given above, while ultimate responsibility for health was attributed by many informants to divine providence, the importance of health information was stressed and inaction when faced with illness was not supported.

Overall, more similarities than differences between three subgroups studied were apparent in the results of our research, although one of these sub-groups was particularly disadvantaged. A cluster of linked perceptions pertaining generally to health and the causes of ill health were found to be prevalent across all the groups studied, and this brings us to a second level of distinctions; that between people of South Asian origin in the UK and those living in South Asia. The perception of bodily health as related to environmental adaptation in which climate, the ingestion of appropriately balanced foodstuffs and activity patterns all play a part, together with the view that individual constitution plays a significant role in determining susceptibility to ill health, was expressed by most of our informants regardless of their particular geographical origins, language or religion. These ideas are strikingly similar to well-documented South Asian 'humoral' conceptions of health (Leslie 1980; Lambert 1992: 1070–1071) which posit an ecological flow of substances and qualities between the environment, food and the human body (Zimmerman 1987). In South Asia, both ingested substances and seasonal conditions are understood to affect individual health. These ideas are related to the humoral theories found in both Ayurveda and Unani Tibb, the main textual traditions of South Asian medicine. In popular discourse (in contrast with indigenous expert medical knowledge), specific health problems are rarely attributed precisely to excesses or deficiencies of specified humours, but the general notion that diet and style of life should be appropriate for the climate in which a person lives in order to maintain bodily health is ubiquitous. Among our informants, conceptions concerning the effects of hot climate and physical activity as conducive to a reduction in body fat were operationalised through a literalist interpretation of the action of sweating. These 'humoral' ideas were also linked in a subtle manner with the recognition of individual differences via the notion of 'constitution'.

Constitution was recognised to be another variable that affects individual susceptibilities to disease and responses to treatment, thus providing a place in lay understanding for the variations that are observed to exist between individuals in their capacities to maintain health under similar conditions. While constitutional make up is seen as inherent (or genetic), individual susceptibilities are also predictably linked to life-cycle stages and particular circumstances. Thus, just as intake of 'cooling' foods should be limited during cold weather, people in states of physical vulnerability should adopt a diet that is appropriately modified to their condition. This principle is the source of the commonly expressed concern to receive advice on dietary modification when taking medication for ill health, since both the condition itself and the medication taken are understood to affect internal bodily state and should therefore be counteracted by appropriate dietary adjustments.

It would be inappropriate, however, to conclude from these findings that 'culture', as expressed in ideas about health, constitutes a static and unchanging body of knowledge. In their accounts of the determinants of ill health, our informants strongly emphasised not only their changed styles of living and eating but also influences such as 'stress' that occupy a prominent place in English popular discourse about the sources of ill health too, and other medically defined risk factors that are emphasised in health education information. These latter attributions did not replace but rather were interwoven with more 'traditional' understandings of the nature of health and influences upon it. Furthermore, 'humoralist' understandings and accounts that emphasise the effects of migration are likely to be more predominant among first-generation immigrants, such as most of our informants, than among British-born people of South Asian origin. Culture in general is made as much as given, and our data suggest a fluid complexity in health-related ideas as new circumstances, information, observations and life events are given meaning and interpreted (Stubbs 1993: 47 argues for the need to move away from understandings of culture as a monolithic entity disconnected from individual experience and from racism and other oppressions). Given both the personal histories of those interviewed, and the emphasis placed in South Asian medical systems and folk ethno-medical notions on the adaptive relationship between person and local environment in maintaining health, it is unsurprising that our informants tended to attribute common health problems experienced by people of South Asian origin to their migration experience. The 'migration effect' has been noted in health-related literature, but discussion generally focuses either on the detrimental effects that the stress of migration may have on health, or on the 'healthy migrant' selection effect of migration. Little attention has been given previously to migrants' own conceptualisations of the effects of migration on their health. Our findings reveal that among South Asian informants, explanations of poor health following migration emphasise problems of adaptation to a different ecological zone and changes in living styles rather than the effects of the migration experience itself.

Some researchers in the field of health and ethnicity have attributed increased rates of specific diseases among certain minority ethnic groups to a failure to 'adapt' to the British way of life (Khan 1979; Goel et al. 1981). While such views as propounded by observers have justifiably been criticised on the grounds that they stigmatise the lifestyles of these minority groups, it is interesting that the notion of 'maladaptation' was a recurrent theme in the explanations for ill health put forward by informants themselves. For people who have migrated from a warm to a cold climate and often into very different occupations and living patterns, an increase in the observed incidence of a particular disease (such as CHD) is, within a pre-existing framework of humoral conceptions, readily attributed to physiological, behavioural and dietary non-adaptation. Indeed, in one study women of South Asian origin who were formerly vegetarian reported starting to eat meat since arriving in the UK (Donovan 1983: 29), an approach consistent with the indigenous categorisation of meat as 'heating' in its effects on the body and thus as appropriate for the maintenance of internal balance in a cold climate.

While the explanatory idiom is one of humoral imbalance and improper digestion, it is interesting that the lay epidemiological explanations of our informants are, with their focus on weight gain and ill health through fat accumulation and lack of exercise, in striking accord with recent epidemiological theories that strive to account for the increased incidence of heart disease among South Asian migrants. A hypothesis favoured by researchers is that of 'insulin resistance', in which a genetic adaptation common among South Asians that enhances the physiological ability to store fat in times of food scarcity leads, in situations of food abundance and lack of physical activity, to insulin resistance, central obesity and increased susceptibility to diabetes and CHD (McKeigue, Shah and Marmot 1991).

Most research on cultural aspects of health confines analysis to the particular group under study and, as discussed previously, in the absence of comparative research among different groups it is difficult to do otherwise. However, a substantial body of material exists on lay concepts of health among white British people both generally and in relation to CHD in particular. Comparison can thus be made between people of South Asian origin and white indigenes. One striking finding of our research into concepts pertaining to the causes and prevention of CHD among people of South Asian origin is that their ideas are rather similar to those of white British people. In many respects – the emphasis on stress, on inheritance and on 'lifestyle' factors such as smoking, drinking and eating the wrong food in attributions of etiology, together with a healthy scepticism about health education messages – our findings concur with those of studies undertaken among native British people in South Wales (Davison, Frankel and Davey Smith 1989, 1992; Davison, Davey Smith and Frankel 1991) and in England (Rose and Lambert 1990; Lambert and Rose, 1996). There seem to be few differences between the native British population in general and the various South Asian sub-groups we studied as far as ideas about susceptibility to CHD, the interpretation of health education messages and the relationships between information and behavioural change are concerned. One reason for this is exposure among both groups to health education information; our research supports other findings (Davison, Davey Smith and Frankel 1991; Kay, Shaikh and Bhopal 1990) which have suggested that health education messages are well known among lay people from a variety of backgrounds, in contrast with Bhopal's (1986) earlier finding.

We suggest, however, that this is not the only, or even the main, reason why perceptions of risk, CHD and health maintenance are similar amongst UK residents of British and of South Asian origin. Other research into lay understandings of health and disease has repeatedly found, in keeping with our study, that such ideas are shaped by the context of everyday experiences (including life circumstances and previous personal and family history) and that health-related behaviour is influenced by practical constraints upon time and resources. When a disease or other health problem is sufficiently common to form part of most people's own experience (whether by directly affecting them or by affecting people known to them), information about it from professional sources can be compared directly with personal knowledge. The 'lay epidemiology' (Davison, Davey Smith and Frankel 1991) of CHD that is acquired through personal knowledge may challenge official representations. For example, recognition of family history (heredity) as an important risk factor for CHD is present in lay understandings among both white British and people of South Asian origin alike, although it is strikingly absent in health education material which gives prominence instead to those 'lifestyle' risk factors that are individually modifiable. This discrepancy between official information and collective experience can lead to scepticism about the former and, in turn, to mistrust of the sources of such information.

Conversely, health education that concords with lay people's views about the causes of ill health may be readily accepted and there is some evidence for this process in our data relating to dietary modification. Emphasis has been placed on diet in the health education materials and campaigns directed at South Asians (Bhatt and Dickinson 1992). This may be the consequence of an earlier focus on rickets, in which dietary changes and supplementation were advocated as a response, or of an erroneous assumption that high levels of fat in the 'traditional' South Asian diet are responsible for the high observed incidence of coronary heart disease (Silman *et al.*

1985). 'Heart health' campaigns directed at people of South Asian origin in London continue to focus prominently on dietary modification as a means of risk reduction. This emphasis may aggravate the tendency, discussed above, of health professionals to construe particular health problems among specific minority ethnic groups as resulting from their 'traditional' lifestyles (that is, their culture). Our findings suggest that the targets of such campaigns have proved highly receptive to these messages. Frequent reference was made by our informants to the unhealthiness of the 'traditional diet' of South Asian people and this is indicative of a process in which the dominant ethnic group's representation of a particular cultural attribute as pathological is 'internalised' by members of the minority group in question. We suggest that these messages are assimilated especially readily because they resonate with pre-existing ideas about the importance of appropriate dietary modification in maintaining health under changed environmental conditions (due to migration). It is particularly unfortunate that attempts to encourage dietary change for disease prevention purposes have focused on aspects of dietary practice such as fat content that, among South Asians, actually need little modification. Among this group these aspects are particularly likely to be emphasised because they dovetail with lay concepts about healthy eating. Meanwhile, few attempts have been made in health promotion initiatives to address other aspects of dietary practice, such as excess intake of food in general (which leads to obesity, a major risk factor for CHD and diabetes), although these could just as easily be couched in terms that would concur with popular understandings, such as the notion that body fat is more readily accumulated in a cold climate. Nor has health education material counterbalanced the message that the traditional South Asian diet is 'bad' by highlighting the protection it appears to afford against other diseases, such as colo-rectal cancer (McKeigue *et al.* 1989a, Matheson *et al.* 1985).

Apart from the contrasts and similarities between different groups, another type of 'difference' is worth examining in our material, particularly given the ways in which the setting of research agendas in the field of ethnicity and health tend to operate. This concerns potential distinctions between disease-specific concepts and general ideas about health. Because of the pre-eminence of the biomedical paradigm in public health and health services research, even qualitative studies into cultural dimensions of health among minority groups tend to be framed by biomedically defined disease categories. Where, as in the studies described here, the purpose of the research is to assist in framing health education or health promotion strategies directed at a particular public health problem, the research focus tends to be confined to the investigation of how the biomedical disease category in question is understood. As a result, the data collected frequently constitute isolated observations, such as 'knowledge' or 'beliefs' about particular health problems. Without reference to the broader, often non-health-specific, cultural constructs, social determinants and individual histories in which such ideas are embedded, these data can be difficult to interpret and often conspire to reinforce assumptions about the apparent irrationality of lay ideas and practices so identified. For example, when taken out of the context of a broad configuration of underlying ethno-medical principles concerning environmental and dietary adaptation and the maintenance of health, combined with awareness of the changes in work, activity and eating patterns consequent upon migration, our informants' statements that hot weather 'melts fat' would appear as a simple misconception. Again, the material presented in this chapter on perceptions of health and ill health suggests that views about the causes and means of prevention of coronary heart disease derive from more general understandings of health and the body as well as from disease-specific constructs derived from health education information and personal familiarity with the disease.

CONCLUSIONS

In conclusion, it is clear that common to all the South Asian groups in our study was a distinctive and subtle configuration of ideas that interrelated individual constitution, diet and climatic conditions to individual health status and prevailing life circumstances in a complex manner. In other respects, our findings did not seem to be strikingly culturally specific either to specific sub-groups in particular or to South Asians in general. One form of variation between the three sub-groups of South Asian origin was noted in relation to the distinctive concerns of Bangladeshis in the first study. However, this observation provides a good illustration both of the difficulties entailed in attempting to determine the core components of ethnicity as a means of identifying and targeting particular 'ethnic groups' and of the dangers inherent in attributing particular perceptions and practices to the 'culture' of any such group. Religiously observant – or poor – Bengali-speaking Muslims, for example, might have more in common with the religiously observant – or poor – of other faiths regardless of their geographical origins in their attitudes to health promotion or their use of health services, than with non-observant – or wealthy – Bengali speakers, whether Hindu or Muslim, Bangladeshi or Indian. In this case, neither religion, nor language, nor country of origin necessarily constitute predictors of how health-related information and advice may be received or responded to, whereas in other respects (such as advice on dietary change) the first two components of identity at least may be relevant indications of the kinds of information likely to be useful to a particular group.

It has not been possible within this chapter to compare our research findings with those concerning health-related ideas among other minority ethnic groups as well as among native British people, but there are indications (see Donovan 1986) that certain themes – such as the view that family and financial worries are a cause of ill health – are held in common with people of Afro-Caribbean origin too. Overall, our informants' perceptions of health, ill health and the causes and prevention of coronary heart disease were more characteristic of the way in which lay people generally interpret illness than of either disease-specific or culturally specific representations. Although the latter were important, culturally specific ideas were just one component in informants' understandings. Health and the occurrence of ill health was interpreted in relation to people's life situation and in the light of knowledge derived from personal and social experience too, and all these elements in turn were brought to bear on the evaluation of health information received from professional sources. Thus, one significant binary contrast in understanding 'cultural differences' in health concepts among minority ethnic groups may be the most obvious, but least often considered in sociological and anthropological studies of ethnicity and health: that between biomedical and a generalised lay 'health culture'.

'Cultural', 'culturalist' (Pearson 1986) or 'cultural sensitivity' (Stubbs 1993: 38–39) approaches in the field of ethnicity, race and health have been broadly criticised on the grounds that in identifying cultural differences as the main problem, they purport to provide a solution – increasing mutual understanding and thereby improving communication – which fails to acknowledge the importance of racism and the fundamental imbalances of power that exist between the majority and minority ethnic groups. While arguing that a focus on 'culture' diverts attention from structural inequalities, however, these critiques do not dispute the 'fact' of cultural difference (Pearson 1986: 105) as systematically correlated with distinctive, bounded ethnicities and thus as relevant to health status and health provision. In this chapter we have suggested that the very existence of 'cultural differences' in health perceptions and responses to disease prevention strategies which predictably correspond to ethnic affiliation needs to be treated as a question to be addressed through empirical investigation rather than taken as a self-evident assumption. Our findings suggest that understanding people's perceptions of health and responses to health information also require attention to dimensions which cross-cut ethnic affiliation, including micro- and macro-historical context and social structural features (such as socio-economic status, education, gender and age).

Such an approach does not exclude a place for efforts to ensure that health services and information are culturally and linguistically appropriate and accessible to those who utilise them. Stubbs observes that:

'Cultural sensitivity and knowledge of naming patterns may well not be the sole answer to the problems of those who find themselves in a society structured by racism and inequality, but they are none the less necessary, for ignorance is one of the key instruments of racist oppression.

(Stubbs 1993: 189)

Most purportedly 'culturally sensitive' approaches to ethnicity in the health field deserve criticism since they are frequently based not on detailed empirical knowledge that reveals the complex interplay of influences which constitute 'culture', but on crude stereotypes; the reification of the culture of minority ethnic groups as static, monolithic entities that can be categorised by an index of stereotypic cultural traits and their associated pathologisation is a consequence of this absence of knowledge.

NOTES

1 'South Asia' refers to the Indian subcontinent (including Pakistan, India, Bangladesh and Sri Lanka). In the UK, people who themselves or whose ancestors migrated from this region are commonly termed 'Asians' in the

medical literature but this is inappropriate, both because 'Asia' is generally employed to designate a much broader geographical region (including East and South East Asia) and because in the USA the term 'Asian' is generally used to refer to people of East Asian origin (including China, Japan, Korea and Vietnam).

2 Nevertheless, a recent Department of Health guide for the NHS on applying *Health of the Nation* targets (Department of Health 1993) is divided into chapters by disease category and, while mentioning the need to develop appropriate campaigns and services on the final page, specifies only 'an urgent need for *epidemiological* research' (ibid.: 54; our emphasis). By contrast, see Bhopal and White (1993: 148–149, 163) and Johnson (1993: 188–189) on the need for information derived from qualitative research in the development of appropriate health promotion and service delivery respectively.

3 For example, in an analysis of health education materials produced for minority communities, Bhatt and Dickenson (1992) note that the provision of such materials in a variety of languages assumes homogeneity for the different linguistic groups. Reporting a study that identifies epidemiological differences in diabetes prevalence (a risk factor for CHD) among sub-groups of Kenyans of Hindu Indian origin, they suggest that 'more finely tuned analysis may be required, and gives further reason for caution when interpreting indicators of provision for minority communities' (ibid.: 76). Yet service providers might regard the resource implications of providing material specifically targeted at, in this example, Gujarati-speaking Jains, Muslims, Patels and Bhatias alone as highly problematic. The degree to which epidemiological differences in risk for a disease reflect and are reflected by cultural differences is a central concern of this chapter.

4 A further possible set of comparisons could be made between people of South Asian origin in the UK and those of other minority ethnicities. Neither space nor sufficient detailed and directly comparative material are available for us to be able to undertake this task systematically, but see the Conclusions for some tentative comments.

REFERENCES

Ahmad, W. I. U. (1989) 'Policies, pills, and political will: a critique of policies to improve the health status of ethnic minorities', *Lancet* 21/1: 148–150.

Ahmad, W. I. U. (ed.) (1992) *The Politics of 'Race' and Health*. Bradford: Race Relations Research Unit.

Ahmad, W. I. U. (ed.) (1993) *'Race' and Health in Contemporary Britain*. Buckingham: Open University Press.

Ahmad, W. I. U., Kernohan, E. E. M. and Baker, M. R. (1989) 'Health of British Asians: a research review', *Community Medicine* 11: 49–56.

Balarajan, R. (1991) 'Ethnic differences in mortality from ischaemic heart disease and cerebrovascular disease in England and Wales', *British Medical Journal* 302: 560–564.

Balarajan, R. and Soni Raleigh, V. (1993) *Ethnicity and Health: A Guide for the NHS.* London: Department of Health.

Bhatt, A. and Dickinson, R. (1992) 'An analysis of health education materials for minority communities by cultural and linguistic group', *Health Education Journal* 51(2): 72–77.

Bhopal, R. S. (1986) 'Asians' knowledge and behaviour on preventive health issues: smoking, alcohol, heart disease, pregnancy, rickets, malaria prophylaxis and surma', *Community Medicine* 8(4): 315–321.

Bhopal, R. S. and White, M. (1993) 'Health promotion for ethnic minorities: past, present and future' in W. I. U. Ahmad (ed.) *'Race' and Health in Contemporary Britain.* Buckingham: Open University Press.

Bowler, I. (1993) ' "They're not the same as us": midwives' stereotypes of South Asian descent maternity patients', *Sociology of Health and Illness* 15(2): 157–178.

Crawford, R. (1977) 'You are dangerous to your health: the ideology and politics of victim blaming', *International Journal of Health Services* 7(4): 663–680.

Davison, C., Davey Smith, G. and Frankel, S. (1991) 'Lay epidemiology and the prevention paradox: the implication of coronary candidacy for health education', *Sociology of Health and Illness* 13(1): 1–19.

Davison, C., Frankel, S. and Davey Smith, G. (1989) 'Inheriting heart trouble: the relevance of common-sense ideas to preventive measures', *Health Education* 4(3): 329–340.

Davison, C., Frankel, S. and Davey Smith, G. (1992) 'The limits of lifestyle: re-assessing "fatalism" in the popular culture of illness prevention', *Social Science and Medicine* 34(6): 675–685.

Department of Health (1993) *The Health of the Nation: A Strategy for Health in England.* London: HMSO.

Donovan, J. (1983) 'Black people's health: a different way forward?', *Radical Community Medicine* 6 (Winter): 20–29.

Donovan, J. (1984) 'Ethnicity and health: a research review', *Social Science and Medicine* 19: 663–670.

Donovan, J. (1986). 'Black people's health: a different approach' in T. Rathwell and D. Phillips (eds) *Health Race and Ethnicity.* London: Croom Helm.

Goel, K. M., Campbell, S., Logan, R. W. *et al.* (1981) 'Reduced prevalence of rickets in Asian children in Glasgow', *Lancet* ii: 405–407.

Janz, N. K. and Becker, M. H. (1984) 'The health belief model: a decade later', *Health Education Quarterly* 2(1): 1–47.

Johnson, M. (1993) 'Equal opportunities in service delivery: responses to a changing population?' in W. Ahmad (ed.) *'Race' and Health in Contemporary Britain.* Buckingham: Open University Press.

Kay, E. J., Shaikh, I. and Bhopal, R. (1990) 'Dental knowledge, beliefs, attitudes and behaviour of the Asian community in Glasgow', *Health Bulletin* 48(2): 73–80.

Khan, V. S. (ed.) (1979) *Minority Families in Britain: Support and Stress.* London: Macmillan.

Lambert, H. (1992) 'The cultural logic of Indian medicine: prognosis and etiology in Rajasthani popular therapeutics', *Social Science and Medicine* 34(10): 1069–1076.

Lambert, H. and Rose, H. (1996) 'Disembodied knowledge? Making sense of medical science' in A. Irwin and B. Wynne (eds) *Misunderstanding Science: Making Sense of Science and Technology within Everyday Life*. Cambridge: Cambridge University Press.

Leslie, C. (1980) *Asian Medical Systems*. Berkeley, CA: University of California Press.

McKeigue, P. and Sevak, L. (1994) *Coronary Heart Disease in South Asian Communities: A Manual for Health Promotion*. London: Health Education Authority.

McKeigue, P. M., Adelstein, A. M., Marmot, M. G. *et al.* (1989a), 'Diet and fecal steroid profile in a South Asian population with a low colon cancer rate', *American Journal of Clinical Nutrition* 50: 151–154.

McKeigue, P. M., Miller, G. J. and Marmot, M. G. (1989b) 'Coronary heart disease in South Asians overseas: a review', *Journal of Clinical Epidemiology* 42(7): 597–609.

McKeigue, P. M., Shah, B. and Marmot, M. G. (1991) 'Relation of central obesity and insulin resistance with high diabetes prevalence and cardiovascular risk in South Asians', *Lancet* 337: 382–386.

McKenzie, K. J. and Crowcroft, N. S. (1994) 'Race, ethnicity, culture, and science: researchers should understand and justify their use of ethnic groupings', *British Medical Journal* 309: 286–287.

Matheson, L. M., Dunnigan, M. G., Hole D. *et al.* (1985) 'Incidence of colo-rectal, breast and lung cancer in a Scottish Asian population', *Health Bulletin* 43(5): 245–249.

Pearson, M. (1986) 'The politics of ethnic minority health studies' in T. Rathwell and D. Phillips (eds) *Health Race and Ethnicity*. London: Croom Helm.

Phillips, D. and Rathwell, T. (1986) 'Ethnicity and health: introduction and definitions' in T. Rathwell and D. Phillips (eds) *Health Race and Ethnicity*. London: Croom Helm.

Pill, R. M. and Stott, N. C. M. (1987) 'The stereotype of working-class "fatalism" and the challenge for primary health care promotion', *Health Education Research* 2(2): 105–114.

Rocheron, Y., Dickinson, R. and Khan, S. (1989) *Evaluation of the Asian Mother and Baby Campaign*. Leicester: Centre for Mass Communication Research, University of Leicester.

Rose, H. and Lambert, H. (1990) *Genetic disorder: Self help, knowledge and dissemination* (report to Economic and Social Research Council).

Rosenstock, I. M. (1974) 'The health belief model and prevention health behaviour', *Health Education Monograph* 2: 354–386.

Senior, P. A. and Bhopal, R. (1994) 'Ethnicity as a variable in epidemiological research', *British Medical Journal* 309: 327–330.

Sevak, L. and Lambert, H. (1994) '*Coronary heart disease prevention among the Gujarati community in Brent*' (report to Kensington, Chelsea, Westminster, Brent and Harrow Health Promotion Unit).

Sevak, L. and McKeigue, P. (1993) '*Health beliefs and heart disease preven-*

tion in South Asian men and women: implications for health promotion (report to the Department of Health).

Silman, A., Loysen, E., De Graff, W. *et al.* (1985) 'High dietary fat intake and cigarette smoking as risk factors for ischaemic heart disease in Bangladeshi male immigrants in East London', *Journal of Epidemiology and Community Health* 39: 301–303.

Stubbs, P. (1993) '"Ethnically sensitive" or "anti-racist"? Models for health research and service delivery', in W. I. U. Ahmad (ed.) *'Race' and Health in Contemporary Britain*. Buckingham: Open University Press.

Townsend, P. and Davidson, N. (1982) *Inequalities in Health: The Black Report*. London: Penguin.

Zimmerman, F. (1987) *The Jungle and the Aroma of Meats: An Ecological Theme in Hindu Medicine*. Berkeley, CA: University of California Press.

Chapter 8

Ethnic origin of sickle and thalassaemia counsellors

Does it matter?

Elizabeth N. Anionwu

INTRODUCTION

> There are good reasons for counselling of ethnic minorities to be
> carried out by members of the communities involved . . . the deli-
> cate matter of ethnically-determined susceptibility to disease
> does not cause problems when counselling is done 'within' the
> group. Finally, the fact that members of ethnic minorities hold
> responsible posts in the medical team sets at rest any anxiety
> about racist overtones.
>
> (Royal College of Physicians 1989: 28)

Since 1979 the National Health Service has witnessed the emergence
of a new body of health professionals, sickle and thalassaemia counsellors. Most are community nurses, predominantly from black and
minority ethnic communities.

It is estimated that the inherited blood conditions of sickle cell
disorders and beta thalassaemia syndromes affect 6,000 people
(Department of Health 1993), the same as the number of people
with cystic fibrosis or haemophilia. One key difference is that the
former conditions, also known as the haemoglobinopathies, mainly
affect black and minority ethnic communities. The legacy of inadequate health care provisions for multi-ethnic populations is well
documented (Ahmad 1992, 1993; Balarajan and Soni Raleigh
1993; Gill and Johnson 1995; Rassool 1995). The needs of those
affected by or at risk of sickle and thalassaemia are no exception, as revealed in a recent report from the Department of
Health:

> It was clear from both oral and written evidence that care for
> patients with haemoglobinopathies, and genetic counselling of

populations at risk, is not always of the highest quality, even where these disorders are frequently seen.

(Department of Health 1993: 9)

The report contained 62 recommendations, many similar to those made by a variety of organisations and individuals over the previous two decades (Crawford 1974; Sickle Cell Society 1981; Prashar, Anionwu and Brozovic 1985; National Association of Health Authorities 1991).

SICKLE CELL DISORDERS

There are no accurate figures for the number of individuals with sickle cell disorders in Britain as no co-ordinated system exists for the confidential gathering of such data (Streetly, Dick and Layton 1993). The rough estimates range from 5,000–6,000 affected individuals (Brozovic 1992; Department of Health 1993). Whilst, as noted before, this is equal to the numbers affected by cystic fibrosis or haemophilia, they are not uniformly distributed around the country. The groups most affected are mainly people of African and Caribbean origin, the majority of whom live in urban areas. However, a significant minority live in other parts of the country, and these people can be neglected. In addition, there will be children fostered in rural areas or attending private schools, university students and those who may be taken ill away from home, perhaps whilst on holiday.

Sickle cell disorders (SCD) are characterised by mild to excruciating episodes of pain. When it becomes intense, admission to hospital is necessary for treatment with extremely strong pain killers such as morphine or pethidine. The painful crisis accounts for over 90 per cent of admissions for those with SCD. Under certain conditions their red blood cells have a tendency to 'sickle', i.e., to change their shape from a doughnut to that of a half-moon. The pain arises when these odd-shaped cells block small blood vessels in areas of the body such as the bones, preventing the release of oxygen to that part of the body. Other problems may include damage to various parts of the body depending upon where the sickling process takes place, such as the spleen, brain (e.g., strokes in early childhood), lungs, hips and eyes. Children from as young as 6 months are extremely vulnerable to serious and life-threatening infections such as pneumonia and meningitis (Serjeant 1992; Department of Health 1993; Embury *et al.* 1994). The disorders are variable, unpredictable and, at times, fatal (Platt *et al.* 1994). Life expectancy has increased through measures such as early diagnosis in the newborn, prophylactic penicillin and parental education about the condition (Vichinsky *et al.* 1988). Treatment includes hydration, analgesia, antibiotics, as well as the possibility of blood transfusions in the event of complications such as strokes, and surgery such as hip replacement (Serjeant 1992; Department of Health 1993; Embury *et al.* 1994). More recent management, which is still the subject of debate, includes bone marrow transplantation (Vermylen *et al.* 1991) and hydroxyurea (Charache *et al.*, 1995).

A recurring theme in the accounts of families and professionals is the perception that some doctors and nurses view affected individuals as 'a problem'. As one nurse commented:

> You get used to them saying 'sicklers, watch out'. Why not trust them? I think it's because you can't see any physical evidence, they [nurses] get suspicious.
>
> (Alleyne and Thomas 1994: 730)

The main source of tension often arises during the assessment and treatment of the severe painful crisis (Ballas 1990; Alleyne and Thomas 1994; France-Dawson, 1994; National Health Service Management Executive 1994). Judging the degree of pain is subjective and therefore open to prejudicial assumptions and stereotyping and this is beginning to be recognised by the professionals. Shapiro and Ballas note that:

> In the English-speaking countries, the majority of people are of African descent, whereas the majority of health care professionals are not. Additionally, significant socio-economic and cultural disparities often exist. Cross-racial and cross-cultural communications have been historically fraught with difficulties. The tensions that permeate our society inevitably affect the very human interactions surrounding the care of patients with pain.
>
> (Shapiro and Ballas 1994: 541)

The experience and views of patients have been sought out by the National Health Service Management Executive:

> To me the most important thing is getting the pain under control and then you can relax and have the drip put in. You can answer questions and you can be examined. But when they want to examine you first, put the drip in and ask all these questions, it is

very difficult. You sometimes lash out at them and they think you are being awkward . . . Every time I come to casualty they always seem to assume that I am a junkie desperate for drugs, which I find very insulting and upsetting.

(National Health Service Management Executive 1994: 17)

The SMAC report acknowledged the paucity of research-based evidence in the present management of sickle pain. It has been reported that patients who are admitted most frequently with painful crises form one of the groups at higher risk of early death (Platt *et al.* 1994). The clinical and molecular aspects of sickle cell disorders appear to have attracted most research funds. The relevance of ethnicity and socio-economic status of affected families in respect to service provision has received more attention in the United States (Hurtig and Viera 1986; Hill 1994; Nash 1994). However, Ahmad and Atkin (in press) have produced a useful review of the pertinent issues within the UK.

The experiences of those affected by sickle cell disorders together with the proposals for improved health services started to feature in British publications from the mid-1970s (Crawford, 1974; Kirby 1977; Anionwu and Beattie 1981; Sickle Cell Society 1981; Prashar, Anionwu and Brozovic 1985; Black and Laws 1986; Murray and May 1988; Anionwu 1993). They clearly set out the way that the needs of affected families have become marginalised within the mainstream health services.

THALASSAEMIA

There are two types of thalassaemia syndrome that result in a severe and fatal anaemia. Alpha thalassaemia affects the unborn baby whereas the severe anaemia of beta thalassaemia commences at age 3–6 months.

Alpha thalassaemia

Up to one in 15 individuals with origins in the Far East (such as China, Hong Kong, Vietnam and Thailand) are at risk of being a healthy carrier of alpha zero thalassaemia trait. If their partner is also a carrier there is then a 25 per cent chance that each of their unborn babies could inherit alpha thalassaemia major (*hydrops fetalis*). The outcome is usually a miscarriage or stillbirth, with the added complication of pre-eclampsia and possible maternal death.

Concern has been expressed about the failure of existing screening services to detect this potentially fatal problem in pregnant women from high-risk ethnic groups (Petrou *et al.* 1992).

Beta thalassaemia

There is a national register for beta thalassaemia syndromes that contains the names of approximately 600 affected individuals, mainly of Mediterranean and Asian origin (Department of Health 1993). The nature of this fatal anaemia requires monthly blood transfusions for life, but this leads to a life-threatening iron overload. In order to prevent this complication, patients are required to take a drug, such as desferrioxamine, which cannot be taken by mouth. It needs to be subcutaneously injected over 8–12 hours, five to seven nights a week using a battery-operated pump. Some individuals, particularly adolescents, have difficulty complying with such demanding treatment and many die of such complications of iron overload as heart or liver failure. The UK Thalassaemia Society has raised a huge amount of money to initiate trials with an oral drug. Other possible problems of the beta thalassaemia syndromes include those affecting the endocrine system (such as diabetes), osteoporosis and infections acquired through blood transfusions such as hepatitis C. (Davies, Modell and Wonke 1993; Department of Health 1993; Jensen and Tuck 1994). Bone marrow transplants have been successfully undertaken on a significant number of patients, particularly in Italy (Lucarelli *et al.* 1990).

Life expectancy has increased but some individuals and their families may experience tremendous stresses in coping with the illness (Modell and Berdoukas 1984; Jennings 1990; Ratip *et al.* 1995). The monthly trips to hospital for blood transfusions can disrupt schooling and employment, particularly if they are not available during the evening or weekend. The lack of designated units means that beds are not always available. Patients may also experience long delays in waiting for doctors to come and put up the blood transfusion. The needs of those who do not speak English is an issue that merits further research. A Punjabi-speaking researcher describes the impact on the Pakistani parents of children with beta thalassaemia major:

> Virtually from the first contact in the homes the meetings became counselling sessions. This was the first opportunity the parents

Table 8.1 Examples of some carrier frequencies of haemoglobinopathies in various ethnic groups

Haemoglobin type	Ethnic group	Estimated carrier frequency	
Beta thalassaemia trait	Cypriots	1 in	7
	Asians	1 in	10–30
	Chinese	1 in	30
	Afro-Caribbeans	1 in	50
	White British	1 in	1,000
Alpha thalassaemia trait	Chinese	1 in	15–30
	Cypriots	1 in	50–100
Sickle cell trait	Afro-Caribbeans	1 in	10
	West Africans	1 in	4
	Cypriots	1 in	100
	Pakistanis, Indians	1 in	100
C trait	Afro-Caribbeans	1 in	30
	Ghanaians	up to 1 in	6
D trait	Pakistanis, Indians	1 in	100
	White British	1 in	1,000

Source: Department of Health (1993)
Note: The above does not include all ethnic groups at risk of haemoglobinopathies; further details contained in the above publication.

had to speak about their child and the disease with someone who
spoke their language, gave them ample time and understood
what they had to say. One of the most striking features during
the initial visits was the isolation of the families due to their lack
of awareness of the disease and of contact with other affected
families.

(Darr 1990: 26)

SCD and thalassaemia can be detected in the unborn and the newborn baby as well as in children and adults. It is also possible to
identify many of those who are healthy carriers. Table 8.1 illustrates
that there will be 17 to 100 times more carriers than individuals
with sickle cell or thalassaemia disorders (Department of Health
1993). Public health and commissioning agencies need to ensure
equity of access to the recommended process of information, together with the option of screening and non-directive genetic counselling in relevant languages (Nuffield Council on Bioethics 1993).
It has been noted that:

Cypriots, Afro-Caribbeans and Africans may have access to a community counselling resource, but few Indians, East African Asians, Chinese, Pakistanis or Bangladeshis are aware of haemoglobin disorders, and most have no access to appropriate counselling.

(Royal College of Physicians 1989: 28)

Whilst there have not been as many accounts relating to those affected by thalassaemia, differences have emerged between the experiences of families of mainly Cypriot origin compared to those originating from Pakistan and India (Modell and Berdoukas 1984; Darr 1990; Anionwu 1993). The experiences of the latter groups have been exacerbated by the inadequate or total lack of services that incorporate interpreting and advocacy provisions. One major area of concern is the attitude of some health professionals towards those who marry a close cousin, as illustrated by the following observation concerning Pakistani families at risk of beta thalassaemia:

Typical comments from health workers were 'Muslim families have a fatalistic attitude and do not take any initiatives, they are not interested in prenatal diagnosis, as it is against their religion – there is no point discussing it, they marry their cousins – if they didn't they wouldn't have genetic problems'.

(Petrou *et al.* 1990: 255)

The impact of these negative judgements is illustrated in the following account:

One mother married to her first cousin confessed to having told the nurse they were unrelated 'because they frown on you and question you if you are married to your first cousin'.

(Darr and Modell 1988: 188)

Modell, in commenting on the inaccurate, sensationalist and prejudicial portrayal of the subject in a television documentary wrote that 'Most public and medical communication on consanguineous marriage is misinformed and prejudiced' (Modell 1990: 1663). There has been minimal research and debate about the impact of both ethnicity and thalassaemia on populations within the UK, with the exception of Darr (1990) and Ahmad and Atkin (in press).

VIEWS ON RESEARCH

Whilst barriers do exist between some professionals and service users, one area of mutual agreement concerns the need for more research into better treatment of sickle cell disorders and thalassaemia. People affected by or involved with caring for those with SCD or thalassaemia recently met to discuss their experiences and views about research (*Consumers for Ethics in Research* 1995). Their comments included:

'Someone I know goes into crisis every few months, and at the hospital has to wait five or six hours for treatment, and longer for a bed. A lot of them will die waiting. We always seem to be going round the same issues and being discriminated against, compared with, say, people with cystic fibrosis. As small groups, we need to come together, but we also need a community behind us, including many people that don't have sickle. We should all stand up and be counted. We musn't sit back talking any more, we must act. How can we improve our own organisations?'

(p. 19)

'I have been asked to join two projects on research into thalassaemia. I felt that I was not given nearly enough information, and that the doctors were putting pressure on me to join. They seem to be so keen to try out something if it is new. When you ask for details, what they tell you is so basic you don't really know what's going on.'

(p. 16)

'Is anyone doing research that looks at attitudes, and at problems of stigma and labelling after testing and diagnosis?'

(p. 15)

'I am worried because I was asked to join in a trial of hydroxyurea. I was reluctant but I felt I was being pressured by my doctor. We've had to struggle so much with everything else, and then we felt put under pressure to take part in research, on top of so many other stresses. No one explained that hydroxyurea is different from urea. (There was an earlier trial of urea in sickle cell in the USA in the 1970s, but it was stopped because in high doses urea has toxic effects due to dehydration). We do want there to be more research, but we don't want to feel forced to take part in it. I felt that I was forced to take part in it. I felt that I was being treated like a guinea pig. The doctor said, 'Your life will be cut short if you don't take part.' I felt he was doing the research for his glory, and I want to know much more about what treatment I am having.'

(p. 15)

'I'm surprised your doctor has heard of hydroxyurea. I've met doctors who've never heard of it, and when I tell them it's used in the USA to treat sickle cell, you can see them trying to turn back your questions, to make you look foolish and to hide their ignorance.'

(p. 15)

The findings of the USA multi-centre study on hydroxyurea concluded:

Hydroxyurea therapy can ameliorate the clinical course of sickle cell anemia in some adults with three or more painful crises per year . . . The beneficial effects of hydroxyurea do not become manifest for several months, and its use must be carefully monitored. The long-term safety of hydroxyurea in patients with sickle cell anemia is uncertain.

(Charache *et al.* 1995: 1317)

The positive and negative aspects of these findings present dilemmas that are encountered with research into many other conditions affecting the general population. An article on hydroxyurea in a black weekly paper highlights the additional concerns of racism:

I think we should give the drug a cautious welcome, but any treatment plan should be done in partnership with patients, researchers and doctors. As most doctors are white and middle class, they think black patients have no brain power. We need more black doctors doing something encouraging for sickle cell patients.

(Butt 1995)

In reviewing the accounts of users, carers and professionals the following issues emerge:

- inadequate funding of services;
- lack of knowledge of various health professionals in the primary health care team and within hospitals;

- problems in accessing information, screening and non-directive genetic counselling, follow-up and support regardless of the decision taken, i.e., acceptance or refusal of prenatal diagnosis;
- inadequate monitoring of the quality of in-service and out-patient care as perceived by families and professionals;
- poor level of funding for research into sickle and thalassaemia compared to other genetic conditions that mainly affect the white populations;
- failure of present research agendas to incorporate the priorities of affected individuals and parents;
- increased burden that families experience due to ethnocentric, negative, patronising or racist attitudes encountered in dealings with health care workers;
- failure to provide information in appropriate languages prior, during and after screening and diagnosis of the trait and the disorder;
- difficulties in obtaining support and information from people who respect the cultural backgrounds of the families.

The latter three points were major reasons influencing the creation of sickle and thalassaemia counselling posts.

HISTORY OF THE FIRST SICKLE AND THALASSAEMIA COUNSELLING POST

In 1979, in an attempt to meet the needs of approximately 100 patients in Brent, Dr Milica Brozovic, the local consultant haematologist and I established the first sickle cell counselling post in Britain (Anionwu 1989). The gaps in service provision had been identified by listening to the experiences of users in the hospital, home and community settings. A common complaint from parents centred on the lack of information about a range of issues from the inheritance of the condition to managing the painful crisis. The overwhelming majority had not been offered any genetic counselling, even though a significant number of mothers had been identified as carriers in pregnancy (Anionwu 1988). In attempting to explore this issue I stumbled across the following ethnocentric statement in a British genetic textbook:

> Sickle-cell anaemia is not of great consequence to us in the context of genetic counselling in the United Kingdom. The sickling

trait and sickle cell anaemia appear to be confined to peoples of African and Eastern origin.

(Stevenson and Davison 1976: 274)

Increased attention is being given to the adequacy of genetic counselling provisions for minority communities, training needs of staff and recruitment of ethnic minorities into the genetic counselling profession in the USA and to a lesser extent in the UK (Punales-Morejon and Rapp 1993; Rapp 1993; Smith *et al.* 1993; Weil and Mittman 1993; Andrews *et al.* 1994; Wang 1994; Chapple and Anionwu in press.) Smith *et al.* (1993) refer to the first survey of the US National Society of Genetic Counsellors (NSGC) which revealed that 93.5 per cent were white and that only 6 per cent were male. In the UK, Farnish (1988) conducted a survey of the members of the Genetic Nurses and Social Workers' Association with a response from 29 (74 per cent). It noted that they were all female but it did not include any details about ethnic origin. The present chairperson of the Association thinks that there are about four non-white genetic counsellors based within three of the Regional Clinical Genetic Units, one Afro-Caribbean and three Asians (Guilbert, P.; personal communication).

My activities at the centre were modelled on the work of sickle cell counsellors that I had met on the West Coast of the USA during the mid-1970s. As a result of political and professional accusations of neglect, Nixon had approved legislation that allocated federal funds to develop a network of comprehensive sickle cell centres (Scott 1983). I visited one in Los Angeles and met Sylvia Lee, an African-American sickle cell clinical nurse practitioner who provided a remarkable support service for local families. Her achievements made a particular impact and, as a black nurse, gave me food for thought about a similar approach that could be adopted in Brent. The local sickle cell foundation provided me with the first opportunity to attend a sickle cell counselling course held in Oakland, California. It was an incredibly exciting period as it allowed me to forget about the apathy that I had encountered in Britain and compare notes with predominantly African-American nurses and social workers. They held strong views that culturally appropriate sickle cell services were more suitably offered by black health workers. Eaton suggested that:

> if you still want to help the minority communities, the best way would be to involve the counsellors who are already in the

minority communities. Enable the appropriate amount of money to go in the training of these persons in the subject of genetic counselling.

(Eaton 1973: 331).

This and subsequent visits to the USA enabled me to discuss the political issues relating to black health care and sickle cell disorders, and significantly influenced my choice of a community development approach in Brent (Anionwu 1988). As a black health worker actively involved with a local and national sickle cell support group I had 'one foot in the community and one foot in the health service'.

It was deemed important that the Sickle Cell Centre be accessible and staffed by counsellors acceptable to the community in terms of ethnicity, specialist knowledge and communication skills.

Soon after the centre opened in 1979 it became clear that the information needs of those at risk of beta thalassaemia had been overlooked. This was noticeable for the significant local Gujarati community, particularly as I was unable to converse in the appropriate language. I also recognised my limited understanding of religious and health beliefs that impinged on issues such as carrier testing, prenatal diagnosis and the option of terminating the pregnancy. This personal experience strengthened my resolve to argue the case for recruitment of staff from diverse cultures represented within the local community. It accorded with the views of Murray *et al.* (1980) concerning the needs of minority groups in respect to prenatal diagnosis:

'Where appropriate, counselling should be offered before and after prenatal diagnosis. Ideally, the recipients should have a choice of counsellors, including persons who are members of the same cultural or religious group, who speak the same language, or who share that group's attitudes towards death, disease, abortion and deformity.'

(Murray *et al.* 1980: 1254)

By 1985 this goal was achieved when funding was obtained for two more counsellors, one of whom was Nina Patel, a Gujarati-speaking health visitor. It was extremely encouraging to see the impact of her activities and the increased use of the centre by various sections of the Asian community. Her departure in the early 1990s elicited the following comment from a mother of Indian origin who runs a thalassaemia support group:

> We desperately need someone . . . a specialist in thalassaemia from the Asian community. With a western person, most of the time is spent trying to explain how it is in our culture. You're suffering because of your child and on top of that you are suffering because of all the cultural issues.
>
> (Potrykus 1993: 241)

In 1986 we produced a poster with the deliberate objective of attracting the interest of black and ethnic groups. This was achieved by featuring the photos of the three counsellors to publicise the existence of African, Caribbean and Asian staff. Funding was obtained from the Brent Race Relations Unit and the poster was widely distributed to locations such as general practices, libraries and community centres.

The philosophy of appointing black and minority staff created considerable discussion and occasional disquiet at the thought that whites were apparently being excluded from such posts. I often wondered whether one cause of this unease was due to the emergence of an articulate group of black professionals who were confident about addressing the issues of ethnicity and racism. Whilst acknowledging these dilemmas, I felt that there was an urgent need to recruit staff who were acceptable to black and minority ethnic groups in order to undertake community education in a variety of settings. Kaback *et al.* (1974) demonstrated the effectiveness of involving the Jewish community in respect to information and screening for Tay–Sachs disease, where up to one in 20 Ashkenazy Jews are healthy carriers for this fatal childhood illness. Their programme involved active dialogue with people such as rabbis and the training of Jewish volunteers to educate the community in venues such as synagogues. Whilst conflicts have developed (Potrykus 1993), there has also been positive acknowledgement of the similar strategy that was initiated for haemoglobinopathies:

> At the Brent Sickle Cell Centre in the UK the approaches to genetic counselling described have been developed, in collaboration with the sickle-cell support associations of the black community. The Centre is now a model and a teaching resource for sickle-cell centres that are being set up in other parts of the country as a result of informed black community pressure.
>
> (World Health Organisation 1988: 20)

CURRENT SITUATION IN ENGLAND AND WALES

Although I left Brent in 1990, I have continued to produce a list of sickle and thalassaemia counsellors from a data-base that provides details of similar posts established since 1979. There are now approximately 50 sickle and thalassaemia counsellors located in over 30 districts in England and Wales.

In 1984 the Runnymede Trust undertook a survey of screening and counselling services in England and Wales (Prashar, Anionwu and Brozovic 1985). By now, there were a total of 10 haemoglobinopathy counsellors employed in seven district health authorities (Brent, City and Hackney, Haringey, Islington, Lambeth, Liverpool and Manchester). A component of the study included a more detailed examination of these services but did not include questions concerning ethnicity of the counsellors.

By 1991 there appeared to be about 23 health authorities in England and Wales that had set up counselling and development posts. Apart from the 1984 study no information was readily available about the nature of these services. The author discussed the idea of a study to explore this with the Sickle and Thalassaemia Association of Counsellors (STAC), who received it favourably. The aim of the survey would be to describe the location, funding, qualifications, views of those presently in post, particularly in respect to the relevance of ethnic origin of staff.

Ethnicity has been described as implying one or more of the following:

> shared origins or social background; shared culture and traditions that are distinctive, maintained between generations, and lead to a sense of identity and group; and a common language or religious tradition. Ethnic boundaries are imprecise and fluid.
>
> (Senior and Bhopal 1994: 329)

It appeared to me that the overwhelming majority of sickle and thalassaemia counsellors were of African-Caribbean descent compared to those of Indian, Pakistani or Bengali origin.

I was particularly interested in:

- obtaining a more accurate picture of ethnic origin and languages spoken by the counsellors;
- ascertaining whether they felt that ethnic origin was relevant for the post; and
- the reasons for their response.

AIM OF STUDY

The aim of the study was to provide a profile of designated haemo-globinopathy counsellors primarily employed within the National Health Service.

CRITERIA FOR INCLUSION INTO STUDY

All individuals designated as haemoglobinopathy counsellors who, on a paid full- or a part-time basis, provide genetic counselling and other activities in relation to sickle cell disorders and/or thalas-saemia. Those working for the voluntary sector were excluded from the study.

SAMPLING SOURCE

This was not a national survey of all health authorities in the UK. The two sources of information about haemoglobinopathy counsellors were:

1 The Sickle and Thalassaemia Association of Counsellors (STAC).
2 The list of haemoglobinopathy counsellors described earlier. The list is updated from sources including those attending specialist courses organised by the author since 1982, STAC, perusal of nursing journals for advertisements of new posts and contact by Health Authorities planning to establish services.

METHODOLOGY

There were two parts to the survey:

1 An individual questionnaire which included questions about qualification, ethnic origin, terms of employment and nature of work.
2 A 'centre' questionnaire sent to the senior or lone post-holder to provide background information about accommodation catch-ment area, patient numbers, etc. The term 'centre' did not necessarily imply designated accommodation from which services are organised, rather the locality in which the counsellor was based.

RESPONSE

Part 1 – individual questionnaires

In January 1992, 41 individual questionnaires were sent out and there was a 100 per cent response. Thirty-four fulfilled the criteria for inclusion into the study and the remaining seven were not included for the following reasons:

- counselling in a voluntary capacity (3);
- did not undertake any counselling (2) (one was a development post and the other was a manager);
- employed as a local authority social worker (1);
- employed full time in another capacity but paid by a voluntary organisation to undertake three hours of counselling a week (1).

Part 2 – 'centre' questionnaires

All 23 'centre' questionnaires were returned. Of these three were not included for reasons set out above.

RESULTS

Background on 'centres'

The following list gives details of the year that haemoglobinopathy counselling services were established in the 20 districts.

1979	Brent (now Parkside)
1982	City and Hackney
	Islington
1984	Camberwell
	Liverpool
	Haringey
1985	Birmingham
	West Lambeth
	South Glamorgan
	Manchester
1986	Waltham Forest
1987	Newham
1988	Nottingham
1989	West Berkshire

1990	Coventry
	Leeds
	Wolverhampton
1991	Greenwich
	Bristol
	South Derby

DETAILS ABOUT INDIVIDUAL COUNSELLORS

Year of appointment

The counsellors had been appointed between 1982 and January 1992, (12 in 1990) with the average length of time in post being three years. Three haemoglobinopathy counsellors had been appointed in January 1992, just before the questionnaire was distributed.

Qualifications

Out of 34 counsellors 31 were Registered General Nurses of whom 22 were additionally qualified as midwives and 17 as health visitors. Of the three who were not qualified nurses, one had completed the training but had not taken the exams, one was an overseas medical graduate and one did not list any qualifications but had a background in social services.

All but two had attended one or more haemoglobinopathy courses ranging from 5 to 15 days, 20 of them at courses organised by the author in Brent between 1982 and 1990. A further 11 had attended courses more recently set up in Lambeth (in 1987) and Haringey (in 1990) both of which are now approved by the English National Nursing Board (ENB). In addition, four had attended the genetic counselling course organised by the author at the Institute of Child Health since 1991 and also ENB approved. General counselling courses had been attended by 12, and six of these courses were accredited by the British Association of Counselling and one by the Royal Society of Arts. In addition, 13 had undertaken some form of teaching course and six had degrees.

Training needs

Respondents were asked to indicate whether they needed to undertake any further essential courses. Four replied in the negative, 18 mentioned one course, 12 two and one person gave details of three courses she wished to attend. The commonest course deemed essential was a general counselling course that was 'recognised, advanced, accredited, and/or at diploma or degree level'.

Type of work undertaken

Out of 34 respondents 15 indicated that they undertook the following range of work:

- take blood;
- counsel people (including pregnant women and their partners via the antenatal clinic) found to be a carrier for any haemoglobin variant (e.g., sickle, α and β thalassaemia);
- counsel individuals and families affected by sickle cell disorders, thalassaemia syndromes and other haemoglobinopathies.

In addition, they attended haemoglobinopathy clinics, undertook home visits and gave regular talks to a variety of professional and lay groups.

Management of haemoglobinopathy counsellors

Out of 34 respondents 26 had a nurse as their most senior manager (22 community, two hospital and one midwifery). Over half (18) were happy with this arrangement and of the remaining eight, four were not, one was ambiguous and three did not give a reply. Of the eight not managed by a nurse, four were ultimately managed by a hospital doctor, one by a management committee and one by the radiology unit. Only the latter was satisfied with this arrangement.

Contact with regional clinical genetic centres

In an attempt to ascertain knowledge of and contact with main-stream genetic services each centre questionnaire asked for the name and location of their regional clinical genetics centre and the frequency of contact. For the first section of this question four centres were unable to give any answer and two gave an incorrect answer. In respect to contact with the regional clinical genetics centre only one centre indicated that it was very frequent and eight had no contact whatsoever. These responses reveal a need for closer contact to ensure that haemoglobinopathy counselling does not become marginalised from mainstream genetic counselling activities. Closer relationships might offer something of benefit to each, judging from the extremely positive evaluations of the multi-ethnic community genetic courses established at the Institute of Child Health (Anionwu 1991 and Chapple and Anionwu in press). The respondents' replies to questions concerning the location of their regional clinical genetics centre and their frequency of contact with the appropriate centre are summarised below.

Knew location (N = 20)

Yes	14
No	4
Incorrect	2

Frequency of contact

Very frequent	1
Occasional	8
Very little	3
None	8

Most satisfying/stressful aspects of work

Each counsellor was asked some open-ended questions, one of which concerned which aspects of their work provided most satisfaction and which the most stress. The results are described below.

Most satisfying aspect of work

Three out of 34 did not reply.
Reasons in order of those most often stated:

- Providing support for clients (17).
  Supporting my regular clients because they haven't had long term support [in their own language] before.
  I like helping my own community and being there for them.
  I feel that I'm helping my community.
- Teaching and raising awareness of the community and the professionals (14). Three additionally mentioned their satisfaction

in the ensuing uptake services – the following quote illustrates this:

> Community education and raising awareness especially within the Asian community re thalassaemia. The positive response and feedback is very encouraging.

- Genetic counselling (11). Eight specifically mentioned genetic counselling of those found to be carriers and four the counselling of pregnant women and their partners.
- Implementing change (6).
- All of it (2).

Most stressful aspects of work

Two out of 34 did not reply.
Reasons in order of those most often stated:

- Inadequate resources (13). Specifically mentioned were lack of clerical support, counsellors, accommodation, training, equipment, accident and emergency and other hospital facilities.
- Poor managerial support (11). This included general lack of support, bureaucracy.
- Dealing with social and financial problems of clients (7). These included financial problems, welfare benefits, housing, employment, child care, prescription charges, lack of good transport to school.
- Racist attitudes within the health service (6).
- Bereavement counselling (6).
- Antenatal, prenatal diagnosis and post-termination of pregnancy counselling (5).
- Breaking bad news to parents of newly diagnosed children (4).
- Sense of helplessness and inadequacy (3).
- Ignorance of health professionals (3).
- None yet (1) (person in post for 10 months).

Ethnic origin

Respondents were asked to describe their ethnic origin and the replies were as follows:

African-Caribbean	18
Black	1
Black American	1
African	6

Asian	4
Mauritian	1
Greek Cypriot	1
White (E. European Jew)	1
White (Caucasian)	1
Total	34

Languages

Of the 34 counsellors 10 were able to counsel in the following language/s, but only four of them in any of the Asian ones.

Asian (includes Hindi, Gujarati, Punjabi, Urdu, Bengali)	4
African (includes Twi, Ga, Yoruba, Igbo)	3
European (French, Greek, Spanish)	3

The following response was obtained when centres were asked whether they had experienced difficulties in obtaining interpreters and for which languages:

Yes	12
No	6
Not stated	2
Total	20

The languages for which centres had experienced difficulties in obtaining interpreters were as follows:

Asian	7
Chinese	5
French	5
Somali	2
African	2
Vietnamese	1

Relevance of ethnic origin of sickle and thalassaemia counsellors

In response to the question of whether ethnic origin is relevant for counsellors, the overwhelming majority (27) answered yes, four said no (one of whom added the proviso 'except for bereavement counselling'), one was not sure and two, who whilst not responding, indicated their ambivalence in the section requesting the reason for their response.

The numbers of those who gave a particular response together with their reasons are set out below.

Yes (27)

- Enhances communication, establishes better rapport (20);
- In order to understand and respect culture, health beliefs, e.g., in respect to genetic counselling (19);
- Language (9);
- Haemoglobinopathies mainly affect people from black and minority ethnic groups (7);
- racism: barriers may exist between white professionals and black and minority clients (5).

Some of the respondents' comments in support of a 'yes' answer are given below:

People always seem very relaxed and identify with someone that they know can understand them and their situation and cultural background. This is always most marked if you were to suddenly change the language you are using to use the persons own mother tongue. You can see the joy and the smile and the type of rapport that follows.

(African)

Better rapport if both of the same ethnic origin. If the counsellor is caucasian there is this sudden barrier 'she would not understand anyway'.

(African-Caribbean)

If the majority of clients are from one particular group, e.g. black, then majority of counsellors should be from that group.

(African-Caribbean)

Many social/psychological and cultural implications of SCD/ thalassaemia that colour counselling process and that should be dealt with and appreciated by whoever undertakes haemoglobinopathy counselling.

(African)

Ideally, choice of counsellor should reflect ethnic mix of population. In areas of low ethnic mix this is perhaps not essential.

(African-Caribbean)

Ethnic origin is always relevant and has an impact on all interactions, needs to be acknowledged, looked at continuously.

(white)

As a professional I would not like to think that ethnic origin of counsellor is relevant. However, from the client's point of view, being of the same ethnic background goes a long way to getting over cultural and racial barriers some of the clients experience as problematic. In saying this counsellors not of the same ethnic origin do have some successful relationships with clients.

(African-Caribbean)

The health service is so racist and seen by black communities as racist, it is important that cultural sensitive issues such as genetic counselling for these disorders is given by someone who can speak the same language, understand and empathise with the community, relate to culture and is seen to relate culture by the individuals being counselled.

(African-Caribbean)

If one counsels a white person who has a haemoglobinopathy one feels that a different approach has to be utilised. I personally feel more relaxed with West Indian clients.

(African-Caribbean)

Unsure (1)

I'm still unsure about this, lone counsellors should probably be of the ethnic group primarily served. But where a centre has more than one counsellor, then the ethnic origin is probably not a key requisite.

(African-Caribbean)

Not answered (2)

Dependent on area of establishment

(African-Caribbean)

A very debatable area, several issues to be taken into consideration, for example individual's attitude, clients to be counselled.

(African-Caribbean)

No (4)

Own experience. I anticipated being less than adequate in my post being 'white British' but have never experienced this (or not for that reason!)

(White)

Haemoglobinopathy traits affect so many different minority groups it is unlikely that everyone counselled will be of the same group as yourself. It is more important that the person is 'sensitive to the needs of clients from minority groups' and treats each client as an individual and does not marginalise or stereotype.

(African-Caribbean)

Not if the counsellor treated the clients with respect and has an understanding of their culture.

(African-Caribbean)

Knowledge, understanding is not relevant to ethnicity – however, in bereavement counselling ethnicity is important due to cultural beliefs.

(Mauritian)

Discussion

Of the sickle and thalassaemia counsellors questioned 32 (94 per cent) come from black and minority ethnic groups. Nearly 80 per cent (27) of all counsellors felt that ethnic origin was relevant to the post.

The justifications for their responses highlight the complexity of this issue. The main reasons for those who answered in the affirmative was that counsellors should reflect, as far as possible, the majority of clients using the service. This would facilitate communication in a non-racist setting in order to convey respect for beliefs and traditions in relation to sickle and thalassaemia disorders. This was reflected in the view that the attitude and experience of the individual counsellor could overcome differences in ethnic backgrounds. The importance of communicating to clients in their own language was also emphasised, together with increased uptake of services by the Asian community in centres where counsellors do speak their mother tongue. It would not be too difficult to measure this outcome as evidence of this kind might help justify to increase the appointment of similar counsellors. As of mid-1994 there are 50 sickle and thalassaemia counsellors employed within 31 districts in England and Wales. A telephone survey conducted in February 1995 and updated with each new appointment shows no change in the proportion of counsellors within each ethnic group and the various languages spoken. With the departure of Nina Patel from Brent there are currently *no* haemoglobinopathy counsellors in the whole of Greater London who can speak any of the Asian languages.

Research should be carried out amongst those families and individuals who are on the receiving end of sickle and thalassaemia counselling services. In addition to establishing their views about preferred ethnicity of counsellors, it would also provide a much needed audit of the service as a whole. It does appear that there is a form of 'apartheid' or separatism in the provision of genetic counselling. The overwhelming majority of sickle and thalassaemia counsellors are from black and minority ethnic groups and work outside of the regional clinical genetic centres. This is in complete contrast to genetic counsellors employed within the mainstream genetic services, who are predominantly white.

This dilemma poses many challenges and requires that traditional genetic counselling adopt the approach of recruiting staff from more ethnic groups, as has occurred in at least three of the regional centres. The Sickle and Thalassaemia Association of Counsellors (STAC) and the Genetic Nurses and Social Workers' Association (GNSWA) are planning to establish greater links.

CONCLUSION

I strongly feel that the ethnic origin of sickle and thalassaemia counsellors *does* matter. Those involved in recruiting candidates to these posts should actively seek out applicants from relevant ethnic groups for their local community. This can be undertaken through ensuring that details of the posts are circulated to relevant organisations and advertised in appropriate ethnic minority media.

An additional justification for this view is the need to show evidence that black and ethnic minorities provide some input into sickle and thalassaemia services, even if the key people controlling budgets, such as purchasers, are mainly white. In reviewing the USA experience Culliton (1972) reported that after a racial incident in 1971 between blacks and whites at the National Institute of Health, the director promised to name a black person as leader of the sickle cell programme (this duty had formally been part of the responsibility of the deputy director, who was white).

However, it is not sufficient to appoint anybody who just happens to 'look' the part and/or happens to speak an Asian language. They need to show evidence that they can identify with the needs and beliefs of affected families and populations at risk and speak the relevant language/s for the locality. It is futile to appoint a person who speaks Gujarati for a predominantly Bengali population. There should be somebody on the interview panel who can conduct part of the session in the appropriate language to ensure that the applicant can communicate fluently in the relevant dialect. Where interpreters and advocates are involved, training should be provided about issues surrounding sickle and thalassaemia.

The issue of ethnicity is an important one that should automatically be taken into account in any recruitment policy in addition to gender, class and disability. This philosophy does not mean total exclusion of white professionals. The comments of Nash (1986) are relevant for both white and non-white professionals involved with both sickle and thalassaemia:

> Ethnicity and race are factors to be considered in the provision of comprehensive care to persons where sickle cell anemia exists. The health care practitioner needs to develop a knowledge of the specific group, which would include customs and traditions, while increasing their awareness of their own ethnicity, race and class value base, and how they may enhance or interfere with respectful treatment.
>
> (Nash 1986: 144)

REFERENCES

Ahmad, W. I. U. (ed.) (1992) *The Politics of 'Race' and Health*. Bradford: University of Bradford and Bradford and Ilkley Community College.

Ahmad, W. I. U. (ed.) (1993) *'Race' and Health in Contemporary Britain*. Buckingham: Open University Press.

Ahmad, W. I. U. and Atkin K. (in press) 'Ethnicity and caring for a disabled child: the case of children with sickle cell or thalassaemia', *British Journal of Social Work*.

Alleyne, J. and Thomas, V. J. (1994) 'The management of sickle cell crisis pain as experienced by patients and their carers', *Journal of Advanced Nursing* 19: 725–732.

Andrews, L. B., Fullarton, J. E., Holtzman, N. A. and Motulsky, A. G. (1994) *Assessing Genetic Risks: Implications for Health and Social Policy*. Washington, National Academy Press.

Anionwu, E. N. (1988) 'Health education and community development for sickle cell disorders in Brent', Institute of Education, University of London, unpublished Ph.D. thesis.

Anionwu, E. N. (1989) 'Running a sickle cell centre: community counselling' in J. K. Cruickshank and D. G. Beever (eds) *Ethnic Factors in Health and Disease*. London: Wright.

Anionwu, E. N. (1991) 'Teaching community genetics', *Nursing* 4(42): 37–38.

Anionwu, E. N. (1993) 'Sickle cell and thalassaemia: community experiences and official response' in W. I. U. Ahmad (ed.) *'Race' and Health in Contemporary Britain*. Buckingham: Open University Press.

Anionwu, E. N. and Beattie, A. (1981) 'Learning to cope with sickle cell disease – a parent's experience', *Nursing Times* 77: 1214–1219.

Balarajan, R. and Soni Raleigh, V. (1993) *Ethnicity and Health: A Guide for the NHS*. London: Department of Health.

Ballas, S. K. (1990) 'Treatment of pain in adults with sickle cell disease', *American Journal of Haematology* 34: 49–54.

Black, J. and Laws, S. (1986) *Living with Sickle Cell Disease: An Inquiry into the Need for Health and Social Service Provision for Sickle Cell Sufferers in Newham*. London: Sickle Cell Society.

Brozovic, M. (1992) 'Sickle cell disease', *Prescribers' Journal* 32: 2.

Butt, K. (1995) 'Sickle cell drug test row', *Weekly Journal* 23/2: 2.

Chapple, J. and Anionwu, E. N. (in press) 'Health needs assessment: genetic services' in S. Rawaf and V. Bahl (eds) *Assessing the Health Needs of People from Ethnic Groups*. London: Royal College of Physicians.

Charache, S., Terrin, M. L., Moore, R. D., Dover, G. J., Barton, F. B., Eckert, S. V., McMahon, R. P., Bonds, D. R. and Investigators of the Multicenter Study of Hydroxyurea in Sickle Cell Anemia (1995) 'Effect of hydroxyurea on the frequency of painful crises in sickle cell anemia', *New England Journal of Medicine* 332: 1317–1322.

Consumers for Ethics in Research (1995) Special issue on sickle cell and thalassaemia 17, Summer edn: 1–20.

Crawford, J. (1974) 'Sickle cell anaemia, action urged', *Race Today*: 8.

Culliton, B. J. (1972) 'Sickle cell anaemia: the route from obscurity to prominence', *Science* 178: 138–142.

Darr, A. (1990) 'The social implications of thalassaemia among Muslims of Pakistani origin in England – family experience and service delivery', University College, University of London, unpublished Ph. D. thesis.

Darr, A. and Modell, B. (1988) 'The frequency of consanguinous marriage among British Pakistanis', *Journal of Medical Genetics* 25: 186–190.

Davies, S. C., Modell, B. and Wonke, B. (1993) 'The haemoglobinopathies: impact upon black and ethnic minority people' in A. Hopkins and V. Bahl (eds) *Access to Health Care for People from Black and Ethnic Minorities*. London: Royal College of Physicians.

Department of Health (1993) *Report of a Working Party of the Standing Medical Advisory Committee on Sickle Cell, Thalassaemia and other Haemoglobinopathies*. London: HMSO.

Eaton, D. (1973) 'Decision-making and the interests of minority groups' in B. Hilton *et al.* (eds) *Ethical Issues in Human Genetics*. New York: Plenum Press.

Embury, S. H., Hebbel, R. P., Mohandas, N. and Steinberg, M. H. (eds) (1994) *Sickle Cell Disease: Basic Principles and Clinical Practice*. New York: Raven Press.

Farnish, S. (1988) 'A developing role in genetic counselling', *Journal of Medical Genetics* 25: 392–395.

France–Dawson, M. (1994) 'Painful crises in sickle cell conditions', *Nursing Standard* 8: 25–28.

Gill, P. S. and Johnson, M. (1995) 'Ethnic monitoring and equity', *British Medical Journal* 310: 890

Hill, S. A. (1994) *Managing Sickle Cell Disease in Low-Income Families.* Philadelphia: Temple University Press.

Hurtig, A. L. and Viera, C. T. (eds) (1986) *Sickle Cell Disease: Psychological and Psychosocial Issues.* Chicago: University of Illinois.

Jennings, P. (1990) 'Thalassaemia: levels of knowledge', *Paediatric Nursing* 2: 22–23.

Jensen, C. E. and Tuck, S. M. (1994) 'Endocrine problems in: b-thalassaemia major', *Contemporary Reviews in Obstetrics and Gynaecology* 6: 133–136.

Kaback, M. M., Zeiger, R. S., Reynolds L. W. and Sonneborn, M. (1974) 'Tay–Sachs disease: a model for the control of recessive genetic disorders' in A. G. Motulsky *et al.* (eds) *Birth Defects.* Amsterdam: Excerpta Medica.

Kirby, J. (1977) 'Sickle cell dilemma', *GP* 34.

Lucarelli, G., Galinberti, M., Polchi, P., Angelucci, E., Baronciani, D., Giardini, C., Politi, P., Durazzi, S. M. T., Muretto, P. and Albertini, F. (1990) 'Bone marrow transplantation in patients with thalassaemia', *New England Journal of Medicine* 322: 417–421.

Modell, B. (1990) 'Consanguineous marriage', *British Medical Journal* 300: 1662–1663.

Modell, B. and Berdoukas, V. (1984) *The Clinical Approach to Thalassaemia.* London: Grune and Stratton.

Murray R. F., Chamberlain, N., Fletcher, J., Hopkins, E., Jackson, R., King, P. A. and Powledge, T. M. (1980) 'Special considerations for minority participation in prenatal diagnosis', *Journal of the American Medical Association* 243 (12): 1254–1256.

Murray, N. and May, A. (1988) 'Painful crises in sickle cell disease – patients' perspectives', *British Medical Journal* 297: 452–454.

Nash, K. B. (1986) 'Ethnicity, race, and the health care delivery system' in A. L. Hurtig and C. T. Viera (eds) *Sickle Cell Disease, Psychological and Psychosocial Issues.* Chicago: University of Illinois.

Nash, K. B. (ed.) (1994) *Psychosocial Aspects of Sickle Cell Disease. Past, Present, and Future Directions of Research.* New York: The Haworth Press.

National Association of Health Authorities (1991) 'Words about action – haemoglobinopathies (sickle cell disorders and thalassaemia)', *Bulletin* 4.

National Health Service Management Executive (1994) *Sickle Cell Anaemia.* London: Department of Health.

Nuffield Council on Bioethics (1993) *Genetic Screening: Ethical Issues.* London: Nuffield Council on Bioethics.

Petrou, M., Brugiatelli, M., Old, J., Hurley, P., Ward, R. H. T., Peng Wong, K., Rodeck, C. and Modell, B. (1992) 'Alpha thalassaemia hydrops fetalis in the UK: the importance of screening pregnant women of Chinese, other South East Asian and Mediterranean extraction for alpha thalassaemia trait', *British Journal of Obstetrics and Gynaecology* 99: 985–989.

Petrou, M., Modell, B., Darr, A., Old, J., Kin, E. I. and Weatherall, D. (1990) 'Antenatal diagnosis: how to deliver a comprehensive service in the United Kingdom', *Annals of the New York Academy of Sciences* 612: 251–263.

Platt, O. S., Brambilla, D. J., Rosse, W. F., Milner, P. F., Castro, O., Steinberg, M. H. and Klug, P. P. (1994) 'Mortality in sickle cell disease – life expectancy and risk factors for early death', *New England Journal of Medicine* 330: 1639–1643.

Potrykus, C. (1993) 'Sickle cell – black counsellors under pressure', *Health Visitor* 66: 239–241.

Prashar, U., Anionwu, E. N. and Brozovic, M. (1985) *Sickle Cell Anaemia – Who Cares?* London: Runnymede Trust.

Punales-Morejon, D. and Rapp R. (1993) 'Ethnocultural diversity and genetic counselling training: the challenges for a twenty-first century', *Journal of Genetic Counselling* 2(3): 155–158.

Rapp, R. (1993) 'Amniocentesis in sociocultural perspective', *Journal of Genetic Counselling* 2(3): 183–196.

Rassool, G. H. (1995) 'The health status and health care of ethno-cultural minorities in the United Kingdom: An agenda for action', *Journal of Advanced Nursing* 21: 199–201.

Ratip, S., Skuse, D., Porter, J., Wonke, B., Yardumian, A. and Modell, B. (1995) 'Psychosocial and clinical burden of thalassaemia intermedia and its implications for prenatal diagnosis', *Archives of Disease in Childhood* 72: 408–412.

Royal College of Physicians (1989) *Prenatal Diagnosis and Genetic Screening. Community and Service Implications.* London: Royal College of Physicians.

Scott, R. B. (1983) 'Historical review of legislative and national initiatives for sickle cell disease', *American Journal of Pediatric Haematology/Oncology* 5: 346–351.

Senior, P. A. and Bhopal, R. (1994) 'Ethnicity as a variable in epidemiological research', *British Medical Journal* 309: 327–330.

Serjeant, G. R. (1992) *Sickle Cell Disease*, (2nd edn). Oxford: Oxford University Press.

Shapiro, B. S. and Ballas, K. B. (1994) 'The acute painful crisis' in S. H. Embury, R. P. Hebbel, N. Mohandas and M. H. Steinberg (eds) (1994) *Sickle Cell Disease: Basic Principles and Clinical Practice.* New York: Raven Press.

Sickle Cell Society (1981) *Sickle Cell Disease – The Need for Improved Services.* London: Sickle Cell Society.

Smith, S. C., Steinberg Warren, N. and Misra, L. (1993) 'Minority recruitment into the genetic counselling profession', *Journal of Genetic Counselling* 2(3): 171–181.

Stevenson, A. C. and Davison, B. C. C. (1976) *Genetic Counselling.* London: Heinemann.

Streetly, A., Dick, M. and Layton, M. (1993) 'Sickle cell disease: the case for co-ordinated information', *British Medical Journal* 306: 1491–1492.

Vermylen, Ch. Cornu, G., Philippe, J., Ninanae, J., Latinne, D., Ferrant, A.,

Michaux, J.L.. and Sokal, G. (1991) 'Bone marrow transplantation in sickle cell anaemia', *Archives of Disease in Childhood* 66: 1195–1198.

Vichinsky, E., Hurst, D., Earles, A., Kleman, K. and Lubin, B. (1988) 'Newborn screening for sickle cell disease: effect on mortality', *Pediatrics* 81: 749–755.

Wang, V. O. (1994) 'Cultural competency in genetic counselling', *Journal of Genetic Counselling* 2(4) 267–277.

Weil, J. and Mittman, I. (1993) 'A teaching framework for cross-cultural genetic counseling', *Journal of Genetic Counselling* 2(3): 159–169.

World Health Organisation (1988) *The Haemoglobinopathies in Europe: A Report on Two WHO Meetings*. Copenhagen: World Health Organisation Regional Office.

Chapter 9

The trouble with culture

Waqar I. U. Ahmad

INTRODUCTION

In this chapter my focus is specifically on the way in which 'culture' is used in research and health and social policy in relation to racial minorities. In the discourses on ethnicity and culture, there is an interplay between the two broad interpretations of culture as resources for life and as civilisation. My argument is not that in considering health, illness and health care of minority ethnic groups culture is not important. It is that stripped of its dynamic social, economic, gender and historical context, culture becomes a rigid and constraining concept which is seen somehow to mechanistically determine peoples' behaviours and actions rather than providing a flexible resource for living, for according meaning to what one feels, experiences and acts to change. Cultural norms provide guidelines for understanding and action, guidelines which are flexible and changing, open to different interpretations across people and across time, structured by gender, class, caste and other contexts, and which are modulated by previous experiences, relationships, resources and priorities. The rigid conception of culture, which all too often is apparent in health research serves a different function, however, it provides a description of people which emphasises their 'cultural' difference and helps to obscure the similarities between broadly defined cultural groups and the diversity within a cultural group.

In writing this chapter I am aware of my own limitations. I have a hybrid background as a researcher, having started off on research work in a department of public health medicine and epidemiology and then researching and teaching in a department of social sciences before joining a unit which researches on aspects of social policy. In my research and writings I have been critical of the crude conceptions of culture which so commonly go unchallenged both in research on 'race' and ethnicity in relation to health, and within the informal culture in the health services. My own perspective has emphasised the importance of considering issues of structural inequalities and racism in the lives of Britain's minority ethnic communities; to me, 'culture' has often been used as a decoy to divert attention away from these factors. My experiences both as a member of a minority ethnic group and as a researcher are important in shaping my views on 'race', ethnicity and health research, and the place of 'culture' within it. In the arguments I develop, I have used examples which are much broader than the traditional confines of the sociology of health and illness. To me this is important in locating a discussion of 'culture' in relation to health and medicine within wider concerns in research and policy on minority ethnic groups.

The chapter considers issues in research on ethnicity; debates around 'race', culture and difference; the importance of contextualising culture in gender and social relations and of recognising diversity and convergence between groups and generations; and policy responses to health needs perceived to be located in cultural difference.

'CULTURE', 'RACE' AND HEALTH RESEARCH

Health and 'race' is such a major industry that it sustains current awareness bulletins, clearing houses for information exchange and numerous general and specialist bibliographies. As several commentators have noted, the priorities in published research neither reflect the concerns of minority ethnic communities nor the major problems in morbidity and mortality, or blockages in service provision (Bhopal 1988; Ahmad 1993). The dominant epidemiological approach to 'race' and health research presents the researcher as an unconcerned, objective scientist pursuing scientific truths about populations in terms of risk markers, differences in morbidity and mortality or in patterns of service use. In this traditional medical scientific approach, supposedly objective pronouncements are made on the basis of carefully collected data to test out particular hypotheses. Within this tradition, reference to racism may be seen as inappropriate; humanity tends to be divided along ethnicity, supposedly the primary category for defining difference, and differences in morbidity, mortality or use of health care would then be explained with reference to cultural differences between 'ethnically distinct groups'. That this is a prized tradition within scientific medicine is illustrated by editorial comments (Carney 1989) in the *British Medical Journal* on two articles on ethnic differences in consultations by Balarajan, Yven and Raleigh (1989) and Gillam *et al.* (1989). Sheldon and Parker (1992) note a variety of simplistic assumptions about 'ethnicity' or 'culture' in these articles.

> For example, in Gillam's paper '"the ethnic classification" adopted . . . combined "race" and nationality. Priority was accorded "race" in the case of east African-born Asian.' This paper also refers to 'native Britons', 'Southern Irish', 'West Indians' and 'Asians' (including those born in East Africa). There is no discussion of what they think is being measured but constant reference is made to 'cultural differences'. In the same issue of the *BMJ*, Balarajan, Yuen and Raleigh analysed data from the General Household Survey and used the categorisations, 'White, West Indian, Indian and Pakistani', although in discussion they refer to the 'Asian population living in Britain', the 'indigenous population' and 'second generation immigrant'.
>
> (Sheldon and Parker 1992: 57)

As Sheldon and Parker (1992) note, these papers use disparate notions of identity, and difference dressed up as 'ethnicity' and 'cultural difference' is discussed as a non-problematic, taken-for-granted reality. The accompanying editorial (Carney 1989) emphasises the need to keep politics out of medical research and offered these articles as exemplars of the prized 'politics-free' and objective epidemiological tradition. He argues that research on ethnic minorities should be 'objective so as not to be construed as having political or racial overtones'.

The health and 'race' literature also addresses differences in terms of a deterministic link between 'cultures' of minority ethnic communities and their morbidity, mortality and health behaviour (e.g., Qureshi 1989; see critique by Ahmad 1993). Most research on health and health care of minority ethnic communities is still conducted by health professionals, and it is expected that minority cultures will structure their needs for and use of health services to suit the needs of professionals. Many commentators are pessimistic about the prospects for a rapid improvement in models of research or greater community involvement in setting research agendas. For example, Sheldon and Parker (1992: 71) argue:

It is unlikely that the health professionals will in the short term be able to adopt a more anti-racist perspective that understands conceptually the way in which the process of racialisation has determined people's or patients' social, economic and epidemiologic location. It is only with this understanding that 'race' can be used to inform and explain rather than to obfuscate and oppress. There is little evidence to indicate that health researchers are developing such an awareness.

Critiques of research in various areas of 'race' and health are provided by, among others, Pearson (1986), Sheldon and Parker (1992), Ahmad (1993) and Sashidharan and Francis (1993).

CULTURE, 'RACE' AND DIFFERENCE

Racism is a dynamic force; its manifestations are manifold, its articulation changes across time and space, and its impact is mediated by a variety of social and structural factors (Donald and Rattansi 1992). An important articulation of racism is through the discourse of culture, defined in rigid and static terms where cultures can be identified as British or 'alien', and on this basis people can be regarded as more or less belonging or deserving. Culture thus becomes a vehicle for defining national identity and citizenship. This is the language of the 'new racism', defined as a form of pseudo-biological culturalism:

> Nations, on this view, are not built out of politics, or economics, but of human nature. It is in our biology, our instinct, to defend our way of life, traditions and customs against outsiders, not because they are inferior, but because they are part of different cultures.
>
> (Barker 1981:23)

And racist discourses concerning minority groups in Britain are reinforced by historical considerations. As Lawrence (1982) notes, the underdevelopment and poverty of 'Third World' countries is viewed not as the outcome of centuries of imperialism and colonial dominance, but as the natural consequence of the cultural and genetic inferiority of black people.

The naturalisation of the difference between these cultures and English culture helps to 'explain' why Asians adhere to 'backward' religions and 'barbaric' customs, it also helps to 'explain' the 'superstitious' and primitive' beliefs and customs of Africans.

(Lawrence 1982: 61)

Contemporary relationships between the West and the 'Third World' mirror these historically unequal relationships.

Such discourses are clear in the pronouncements of New Right writers. Husband (1991) argues that stereotypes which link behavioural characteristics with 'racial' or cultural origin are exemplified in the writings of new right thinkers who argue that West Indians are by culture resentful of authority, have an unsatisfactory family structure, low educational standards and involvement in drugs and violent crime whilst, on the other hand, Indians are industrious and peaceful but are profoundly culturally different and have loyalties with the country of origin – they therefore cannot stake a convincing claim to being British (Husband 1991: 61). Since the 'Rushdie affair' and the Gulf War, in Britain, and more widely in Europe, Muslims have acquired the status of being uniquely alien, a group who, because of their 'intolerance' and 'fanaticism' and their treacherous aversion to 'the British way of life' pose a unique threat to good 'race relations'. This perception is itself built upon the ideological foundation of 'orientalism' within the European peoples' construction of their identity in opposition to exotic 'Others'. The pronouncements about the 'natural fear' of ordinary British people about being swamped by alien cultures; minorities proving or disproving their Britishness by their performance on the 'cricket test' or by the strength of their support for 'our lads' in military adventures in the Falklands or the Gulf; lessons to the British Muslims, following the Rushdie affair, on how to be British – are some of the manifestations of the new or cultural racism. Protests against halal meat have been conducted behind the facade of British public concerns for animal rights in Britain. Establishing places of worship, such as temples, mosques or gurdawaras, has been opposed on the grounds of noise, traffic congestion or on the pretence of protecting buildings of historical interest from conversion (Eade 1989), but they could all equally well be seen as examples of protecting the mythical 'British' culture from the threatening 'Other'.

At the time of writing, schools in France are banning Muslim girls from wearing headscarves on the pretext that the wearing of a headscarf is oppressive to women. In Britain, oppression of women in Asian cultures remains a popular subject for British newspapers, where gender inequalities are given a peculiarly 'Asian' slant. Yasmin Alibhai-Brown considers these popular concerns as expressed in the British media:

> Here we are, so the stories go, pathetic Asian women, hurled into hellish pits by our vicious fathers and many brothers, there to dwell with our even more beastly husbands . . . Look at the recently publicised cases of women who kill their partners after years of abuse. Inevitably, when it involved an Asian woman – Karanjeet Alluwalia – the focus was on the accursed arranged marriage. Just a few weeks after Alluwalia's trial, there were two equally horrific stories of white women driven to murder, one of whom had suffered hideous mutilation for ten years. I do not recall headlines screaming 'Love Marriage Horror for White British Woman'.
>
> (Alibhai-Brown 1993: 28)

This debate has powerful historical parallels. For example, Lord Cromer, a staunch opponent of the suffragette movement in Britain stressed the importance of continued colonial presence in Egypt in terms of its liberalising impact on Muslim women while at the same time opposing the efforts of Muslim educational charities towards universal education of girls as well as boys (Ahmed 1992). In relation to India, Brah (1992) notes that the British Raj was legitimised by appeals to the 'civilising mission' of the West which constructed Indian cultures as inferior, barbaric, superstitious and emotional rather than rational or objective. The notions of the Indian 'family' as deviant and the representation of Indian women as 'ruthlessly oppressed creatures who must be saved from their degradation' were central to this discourse (Brah 1992: 69).

Discourses built around the concept of culture and cultural difference play an important part within the strategies of control of black people's lives through state systems of immigration control, education, professional ideologies and practices. The application of cultural or 'new' racism, alongside other forms of racism – at the individual and institutional levels – in health and social welfare is well established (Mercer 1986; Dominelli 1988; Williams 1989; Ahmad 1993). In the guise of cultural understanding one is frequently offered a catalogue of checklists of cultural stereotypes which are regarded as essential characteristics of particular cultural-/racial types and which signify the deviance and peculiarities of minority cultures to the normality of the 'British culture' (Qureshi 1989; Rack 1990).

What is pursued through an adherence to an essentialist notion of culture, with its simplicity and rigidity, is a politics of victim blaming which constructs minority communities as dangerous to their own health. To save them, it is necessary to save them from their own cultures which shackle their minds, their beliefs and their behaviour; their problems are located in their difference; their salvation is in being more like 'us'. A view of culture as a source of nurturing and strength, as providing alternatives to oppressive state systems or mobilising family and community resources to fight racism and disadvantage (e.g., the 'pardoner' system to buy houses), as providing essential tools for resisting oppression, is nowhere to be seen in such constructs. Mercer (1986) notes:

A concern with the psychological dimension of ethnicity is a central feature of the formation of discourses in education, social work, youth services, counselling, and personal social services, which all address themselves to issues concerning 'race' through the culturalist system of representation of difference.

(Mercer 1986: 43)

For effective and improved health care provision, then, the solution supposedly is to equip health and social services providers with the necessary tools of cultural understanding while at the same time resocialising the culturally deviant through health education on the 'proper' use of health services. The Stop Rickets Campaign and the Asian Mother and Baby Campaign may be seen as examples of such resocialisation (Rocheron 1988). The effect of an emphasis entirely on cultural difference to explain inequalities and differences in health status or use of health care services is to pathologise 'culture', making it the cause of as well as the solution to inequalities in health and health care (Mercer 1986; Ahmad 1993).

PROFESSIONAL IDEOLOGY AS A MEDIATOR OF RACISM

Professional ideologies reinforce (perhaps even construct) the dominant notions of normalcy and, as main arbiters of definitions of and solutions to problems in health and social services, act as potent mechanisms for social control. Although under challenge from increasing consumerism and managerialism, and some blurring of boundaries between professional and lay knowledge in health and social services, medical and professional power remains an important tool for exerting social control by allowing the exercise of racist power through the hierarchical relationship between practitioners and patients and between service providers and the users. This happens in psychiatry, general practice, community health services, obstetrics and social work as well as other fields (Dominelli 1988; Fernando 1991; Ahmad 1993; Bowler 1993).

Professional ideologies and institutional practices play an important role in reinforcing and constructing norms. For example, Beveridge's notion of the normal family based on traditional middle-class gender roles has shaped the delivery of state welfare. This white, married and middle-class notion of normalcy is imposed on white working classes as well as minority ethnic communities. For example, in the case of African-Caribbean women, the needs of the British labour market resulted in the migration of women without children in order to fill vacancies in the caring and service sectors. Subsequently, this single status, encouraged initially by the immigration process, has legitimised the pathologisation of the black family (Williams 1996). Ideas about deviant motherhood are also apparent in relation to Asian women. Thus, in the 1970s and 1980s, when the Asian communities were facing an epidemic of coronary heart disease, the major focus of official health education was on birth control and family planning (Bhopal and White 1993).

For the white population, the fallacy of the individualistic and culture-centred approach to health promotion, located largely in the 'culture of poverty' thesis, is increasingly being challenged (Research Unit in Health and Behavioural Change 1989), although critiques of the culture-blaming emphasis in health education are not new (Crawford 1977). The conception of culture in health research has been criticised for stripping the concept of its complexity and holism and reducing it to 'lifestyle' (Crawford 1977; Phillimore 1989). Phillimore notes: 'In addition to culture as lifestyle we find spectacle too. What the processes have in common, is that each of these versions of culture can be treated as commodities' (cited in Sheldon and Parker 1992). Among proponents of critical public health and health promotion, the importance of locating people's health beliefs and behaviours in their social, material, gender and racial context is well recognised – the *International Journal of Health Services* and *Critical Public Health* provide good examples of this approach. These are important factors in shaping culture and structuring choices as well as constraints; and people's different locations on these axes impact on their cultural beliefs and behaviours, their ability to affect and challenge the dominant norms and, over time, to make the fit between 'traditional norms and social reality closer.

'RACE', 'CULTURE' AND THE STATE

That the state welfare system oppresses black people is not surprising. The historical cast of the British welfare state rests in large part on racist and eugenicist grounds. Fears about the future of the 'British race' and the loss of the empire; concerns about men's fitness for war and women's fitness for motherhood; threats of the 'unfit classes' – the working classes, 'moral and mental imbeciles' and immigrants – contaminating the thrifty and productive middle classes were central to the introduction of the welfare state. Many of the architects of the welfare state were prominent members of the eugenics movement (Williams 1996).

In relation to minority ethnic communities, the state continues to play an important role in shifting the emphasis from structure, power and racism to culture, ethnicity and difference. Sivanandan (1991) argues that the wider black unity of the 1950s and 1960s was seen as a threat by the state. Various state policies and agencies therefore attempted to incorporate issues concerning minority groups into bureaucratised social policy with the aim of depoliticising black struggles and disuniting the ethnically and socially contoured but politically more cohesive black alliance. In a speech to a social work audience, he argued:

> So they [the state] had to deconstitute Black, break down black into its constituent parts: Asian, Afro-Caribbean, African – and within Afro-Caribbean, St. Lucian, Trinidadian, African – and within Asian – Pakistan, India, Bangladesh, within that the Gujeratis, Muslims, all sorts of classifications and re-classifications, Sikhs, Sri Lankans, Tamils, the lot . . . After breaking down blacks into their cultures, you give them handouts . . . [through] Urban Aid . . . Section 11 and all the other local authority grants that followed . . . So . . . instead of becoming responsive to our black brothers and sisters we became responsive to the system that gave us the money.
>
> (Sivanandan, 1991: 40)

Although this vision of political unity may itself be a fiction, the official responses did lead to reshaping politically common demands into ethnically distinct needs. In turn, meeting the 'ethnic-specific' needs of 'ethnically distinct communities' through specific projects and initiatives targeted at the level of thus-defined groups has represented a fictive unity of perspectives, needs and values among communities (Watters 1996). The communities in turn have reinforced these constructions through using state systems of support for day centres and 'special projects' organised around the notion of distinctive and culturally cohesive communities. Such fictive unities are also used as forms of resistance to external hostility. Afshar (1994) notes that, following the hostility against Muslims generated in the aftermath of the Rushdie affair and Gulf War, 'there has been a tendency amongst the embattled Muslims in the city and the region to claim a unitary identity and postulate a cohesion of views and values that they do not necessarily adhere to in practice' (Afshar 1994: 144). Yet the diversity of perspectives, and need, within cultural groups is hard to miss. This is something to which I return later.

The ethnic school of 'race relations' gave some credibility to the reduction of complex intergroup phenomena to crude notions of culture and, according to Husband (1991), notions of cultural lag and deprivation, previously applied to ex-colonies and colonies, were easily transferred to explain the situation of black people in Britain. 'The reduction of the complexities of the politics of "race" ... to the simplicities of "culture clash" was perverse but convenient form of analysis' (1991: 64). 'Culture conflict' between minority and majority cultures, as well as between the 'oppressive' and 'imported' cultures of the first generation and the presumably more 'civilised' perspectives of the second generation, was a major theme of writings and research in the 1970s (e.g., Watson, 1977). At the same time, the multicultural orthodoxy, according to Sivanandan, transformed minority cultures into commodities for general consumption – what has been called the 'saris, samosas and steelbands' approach to minority cultures (Sivanandan 1991).

The world of culture and medicine in relation to minority ethnic communities is largely the world of these lifeless, limp, cellophane-wrapped and neatly tagged cultures, rather than one of living and lived in cultures with all their vitality, complexity, complementarities and contradictions, cultures that are empowering, changing, challenging and flexible – cultures that are real. Dodge (1969), Qureshi (1989), Healey and Aslam (1990) and Rack (1990) are among a long list of cultural merchants. There is no shortage of examples of this approach; Watters 1996 illustrates this with reference to Rack (one-time consultant psychiatrist in Bradford). Rack notes the psychiatric problems of Asian women thus:

> Asian women whose days are spent in loneliness and social isolation, cut off from family and social networks. Many older Asian women speak little or no English. Some are confined to their home, by their husbands or by their own timidity, and are seldom seen; others may become surgery-haunters – perhaps because a visit to the doctor is one of the few opportunities for a culturally sanctioned outing.
>
> (Rack, 1990: 290)

The primacy of 'culture' or 'ethnicity' as the primary categorisation of social identity may be reinforced with the adoption of the ethnic question in the 1991 census, and the incorporation of the question into the minimum data-set requirements in the NHS. As Ahmad and Sheldon (1993) acknowledge, 'ethnic' data can serve a useful policy purpose in health and social services, provided the researchers and policy-makers have asked themselves the fundamental question of what information they need and what aspects of cultural identity (diet, language, religion, etc.) are important factors for investigation or policy formulation. For ethnic data to be useful at the local level, 'ethnicity' needs to be defined according to local circumstances; this is what the standardisation will work against. Ahmad and Sheldon note:

> the standardization of such categories will give them a spurious air of validity, as 'natural', 'objective' and 'universal' entities. We consider such potential reification of these categories to be of more than academic significance. One of us has written on the increased racialization of research, with particular reference to health, which has done little to improve service delivery, or to advance aetiological understanding (Sheldon and Parker, 1992). We fear that the availability of routine 'ethnic data' from the Census and its adoption in the NHS 'minimum data set' will give increased impetus to this mindless empiricism. [Furthermore,] such categories may lead to the perpetuation of racial stereotypes of the needs, behaviours and expectations of 'Pakistanis', 'Indians', 'Black Africans', and so on, as homogeneous wholes.
>
> (Ahmad and Sheldon, 1993: 129)

Wright (1983), Ahmad, Baker and Kernohan (1991) and Bowler (1993) have reported on health professionals' negative stereotypes of minority ethnic group patients. Findings from Wright's (1983) study of general practitioners were confirmed by Ahmad, Baker and Kernohan (1991: 54)

> the clear picture to emerge was that General Practitioners held less positive attitudes towards Asian patients. Consultations with Asians were felt to be less satisfying, they were thought to require longer consultations, to be less compliant, and perceived to make excessive use of health care, including visits for 'trivial' and 'minor' reasons.

In a recent study of midwives' perceptions of Asian (largely Pakistani) women, Bowler (1993) notes that the midwives' stereotypes had four main themes: difficulty of communication; abuse of service and lack of compliance; tendency to 'make a fuss about nothing'; and lack of 'normal maternal instincts. Perceptions of certain ethnic groups having high or low thresholds for pain, or Asian women's 'plenty pain syndrome', are discussed by Kushnick (1988). Professional perspectives on minority cultures both reflect and legitimise popular discourses on culture, difference and citizenship and are important mediators of access to substantive rights of citizenship.

THE TROUBLE WITH 'CULTURE'

Colonial history has left its marks so that the cultures of the oppressors have influenced, and themselves been influenced by, the cultures of the oppressed. Most African, Latin American and Asian ex-colonies still have European laws; many have adopted European systems of governance; European languages and educational systems dominate in these countries; and biomedicine has captured the dominant place in defining health and illness and the delivery of health care. To illustrate the hegemony of biomedicine, the resources spent annually on a single medical college in Pakistan are greater than the total resources reserved to promote the major indigenous system of health care, *hikmat* (for a discussion of *hikmat* in relation to Western medicine, see Ahmad 1992), and homeopathy and other approaches to health care. The elite of these countries maintain the *status quo*, and thus their own privileged position. In Pakistan, for example, to be educated is to be able to speak, read and write English, the language not just of the colonial ex-masters but also of the current-day ruling classes. The absurd spectacle of the head of state and ministers of government addressing the nation in English, in a country where more than half do not have access to basic education and less than 10 per cent would be able to understand English, continues. It was only in the early 1980s that Urdu gained recognition as the second official language along-side English. To give an example from another continent, in *The Racism of Psychology* (Howitt and Owusu-Bempah 1994) the African co-author's (OB) childhood experiences in Ghana are recounted:

> In school he sang the British national anthem, God Save the Queen. Geography, history, literature and the rest were all Euro-pean. All subjects, including Greek, Greek mythology, Latin and French, were taught in English and he was encouraged to adopt French as his second language, following English. The language he spoke at home was forbidden; even Asante folk-stories had to be told in English. As with generations before him, he was indoc-trinated to serve all things European, to reject Africa and its culture – to talk, dress, dream, think and eat European.
>
> (Howitt and Owusu-Bempah, 1994: 2)

There are two points worth making here. One is that because of the history of colonialism, and the continued unequal relationship be-tween the ex-masters and the people of the ex-colonies, the cultures of white (colonial powers) and black (colonised) people do not meet on equal terms. 'Cultural difference' and the presumed inferiority of the cultures of the colonised acted both as a major legitimisation for colonisation and for the 'reforms' in the colonised countries. Second, through this prolonged system of external domination, many aspects of the cultures of the rulers and the ruled are charac-terised by similarities rather than difference; however, the relative value accorded to particular cultural norms is often more a conse-quence of power dynamics than of the intrinsic merit of the norms themselves. And differences between ethnic minority groups and the white English middle classes are still likely to be seen as differences between the 'civilised' and the 'uncivilised'.

A startling truth in any rudimentary study of culture, norms and behaviours, however, is the diversity of beliefs and behaviours within a group on the one hand, and, on the other, the convergence between beliefs and customs across cultural groups and across coun-tries and continents. Diversity, after all, is not surprising. Populations of all countries contain among them differences of gender, class and other status markers; in many there are additional differences of language, religion, caste, customs, history, tradition, colour and ethnicity. In the sections below, I make broad points about cultural differences and similarities; the social, economic and gender context of culture; and cultural change.

Cultures: similarities and differences

I wish to make three points here. First, that the notion that we structure our behaviour according to our culturally based health beliefs in a direct and linear fashion is a fiction. Second, that there are marked 'cultural' differences between people defined as part of a cultural group. And, finally, that there is a large degree of convergence between the health beliefs and behaviour of different ethnic groups, even across countries and continents. I will consider these in turn.

Individual beliefs and behaviour

First, to illustrate that individuals do not behave in the fashion of culturally programmed automatons, I will use evidence on patients' choice of practitioners. There is a growing body of literature on the process of selecting health practitioners according to, among other factors, personal beliefs, characteristics of the practitioner, the assessment of ailment and the expected nature of practitioner–patient interaction, and cost and accessibility. Nichter (1980) discusses the relationship of people's perceptions of different types of medical systems, in South India, to their choice of practitioner. As Western medicine was considered 'hot' and 'powerful' its use was avoided for children. When used for adults its 'hot' effects were counterbalanced, after recovery, by using 'neutralising' Ayurvedic remedies. Kleinman and Sung (1979) show that selection also relates to patients choosing the system of medicine to match particular symptoms or illnesses. In the British context, many writers have commented on the Asian women's expressed preference for women doctors (e.g., McAvoy and Raza 1988) without examining consulting behaviour. My own work showed that expressed preference did not relate to consultation with a female doctor (Ahmad, Kernohan and Baker 1989). The disparity was most marked for those Asian women who were not fluent speakers of English; these women were more likely to consult the Asian male doctor. (This practice had an Asian male GP, fluent in the main Asian languages and a white female doctor.)

Cultural groups and diversity

Cultural groups are characterised by diversity rather than uniformity with culture providing (usually) both broad and flexible boundaries for beliefs and actions. I have already noted the diversity in populations defined at the level of 'Indian' or 'Afro-Caribbean'. Further aspects of cultural polarisation are represented by status, urban or rural background, caste, occupation, and so on. Let me illustrate the divergence with reference to two examples. My first example relates to childbirth in Pakistan, which I will illustrate with the aid of three stories from my own observations. It is easy to think of a single Pakistani culture around pregnancy and childbirth, indeed, literature on maternity and ethnicity would support such a view at the level of 'Asian' women (Rocheron 1988). The first concerns an upper-class and educated woman in a metropolitan city in Pakistan who, during her pregnancy, is cared for as a private patient by a prominent obstetrician. Her care is highly medicalised and in many ways is no different from what a woman of similar standing might receive in Britain or elsewhere. She realises that the expected delivery date clashes with her brother's wedding, an event to which she has long looked forward. After discussion with her consultant and various tests, she has an induced birth about three weeks before the expected delivery date (and the wedding). This gives her sufficient time to get into shape for her several sets of designer clothing and play a full part in the festivities around the wedding. She has considerable help in looking after the baby from her 'extended' family as well as domestic servants.

The second story is of a village woman who is cared for by the *dai* (the traditional birth attendant without any biomedical training), who also supervises the birth. A number of women from her family are involved in her care during the pregnancy and birth, and the care is very much in terms of local, folk models of pregnancy, women's health and childbirth.

After childbirth, the woman observes the range of prescriptions and proscriptions associated with the 40-day recuperation period, *chilla* (which bears strong similarities to the Chinese tradition of 'doing the month', see Pillsbury 1978).

The third story, concerns a woman who, with her family, provides hard physical labour on road construction. She works until a couple of days before giving birth and gradually comes back to work a few days after the birth. Although she and her family recognise the importance of the *chilla*, their economic situation does not allow them the luxury of 40 days of rest for a productive earner. As she works on the road, carrying and spreading bucketfuls of hardcore to prepare the road surface, her baby rests in a makeshift hammock strung between two poles stuck into the ground on the roadside. All three are Muslim women in present-day Pakistan, but their lives are differentiated by social class, rural–urban split and access to health care; all three are part of the Pakistani culture and tradition on pregnancy and childbirth.

The second example relates to social construction of mental illness among the Bangladeshis in Tower Hamlets. John Eade (1995) shows that a number of constructions of mental illness are held in parallel. These constructions show flexibility and overlap and they range from notions of possession by jinn and *bhuta* to ideas about distress and trauma, and explanations which fit with folk models of health and illness. Eade classifies these as three discrete but overlapping belief systems – Islamic, medical and folk. In Islamic models Eade combines a variety of religious and spiritual discourses along with beliefs based in ideas about health and illness in formal *hikmat*. Moreover, the construction of mental illness is disputed not just at these broad levels. Within the Islamic discourses are the views of the Deobandis and the Barelvis: the latter sect allow exorcism and spiritual guidance from *pirs* (spiritual leaders and healers), practices the former (conservative) group would regard as un-Islamic.

Both groups would regard belief in possession of jinn (a life-form to which, along with the angels, the Qur'ān makes numerous references) as Islamic but possession by *bhuta* (malicious spirits of dead people) as un-Islamic. What is interesting about the diversity of perspectives on mental illness among the Bangladeshi community in Tower Hamlets is that this is a more homogenous community (in terms of rural background, relatively recent migrants, etc.) than the much more heterogenous Asian communities such as the Pakistanis or the Indians.

Commonalities between cultures

A further issue which makes it difficult to regard cultural norms or practices as peculiar to a particular ethnic group is the degree of convergence or commonality between groups. Evidence for this can be offered from different times as well as different localities. For example, Leila Ahmed (1992) discusses the cultural similarities between Christians, Jews and Muslims in eighteenth- and nineteenth-century Egypt in terms of the high value placed on female virginity at the time of marriage. Also the practice of clitoridectomy in contemporary Egypt is equally strong among the Muslims and the Christians.

A study of two Christian sects by Fuller (1991), in present-day Kerala, South India, provides a fascinating account of both diversity and convergence within and across cultural/religious/status groups. The old-established Syrian Christians occupy a high status in Kerala, a status equivalent to the Brahmins (high-caste Hindus) and high-status Muslims. This contrasts with the Latin or New Christians, mainly low-caste Hindus converted during the British Raj. The two Christian sects remain socially isolated from each other; there is little in the way of socialising, common prayers or intermarriage, largely because the Syrian Christians regard the Latin Christians as the Brahmins regard the 'Untouchables'. To take the example of marriage, Fuller notes that the Syrian grouping is largely endogamous and there are fewer marriages between the two Christian sects than between members of the Syrian Christian group and Brahmins:

> there are [virtually] no marital unions between the Syrians and Latin Christians as marriage would be as unthinkable for a Syrian as would a marriage to a Harijan for a Nayar. Indeed, I have more than once heard it said by a Syrian that it would be preferable for one of their community to marry a Nayar or another high-caste Hindu than to marry a New Christian ... What would happen if a Syrian and a New Christian did wish to marry was regarded by most informants as so hypothetical a question that they could not answer it; it had never happened so far as they knew. But they thought that the priest would probably succeed in persuading such a couple to abandon the proposal.
>
> (Fuller, 1991: 198)

Caste, then is as important a factor in the lives of Syrian Christians and the Latin Christians as it is for Hindus, not just concerning social status but also rules about pollution, its avoidance and neutralisation. Both this and the Egyptian example show the impor-

tance of recognising the overlap between cultural/religious traditions. A similar impact of Hindu traditions is apparent in the
hierarchical caste system among Muslims in the Indian subcontinent. Interestingly, Modood, Beishon and Virdee (1994) note
that for many Hindus and Sikhs in Britain, the strict caste heir-
archies are being replaced by social class as a more appropriate
marker of social status for considerations such as marriage. However, as Thomas (1992) argues, social norms can continue to
exert influence long after the conditions which supported them
have changed.

I have already discussed the diversity of perspectives on mental
health among the Bangladeshi origin population in Tower Hamlets,
as noted by Eade (1995). I will elaborate on the role of pirs in
mental illness, this time to emphasise the similarities between their
discourse and some modern Western discourses on mental illness.
Kakar (1982) considers the role of a pir specialising in mental illness at some length. The notion of possession is central to the
demonological view of mental disorder treated by pirs through the
use of *ilm-e-ruhani* (soul or divine knowledge). 'Demons' may come
in several forms, jinn, *bhuta*, *bala*, etc. In addition to dealing with
spirit possession, pirs also often deal with psychiatric and physical
illness believed to be related to *jadu* (malevolent or 'black' magic).
Kakar, a Western-trained psychologist and psychoanalyst, notes
considerable similarities in the demonological and the psychological
discourses on mental illness: 'To me the balas [malevolent spirits]
are the reification of certain unconscious fantasies of men and
women which provoke strong anxiety in the Indian cultural setting
(Kakar 1982: 29). He emphasises the importance of social,
economic and religious cultural context in understanding mental
illness:

> For if your view is demonological and peopled with 'ghoulies,
> and ghosties and long leggety beasties and things that go bump
> in the night', then any talk of buried feelings is irrelevant and
> certainly very irreverent. Conversely, if one's framework is psy-
> chological with unconscious wishes and fears swirling around in
> a subterranean cavern filled with childhood images of parents
> and siblings, then talk of balas and other demons is patently
> absurd and, well, a little 'crazy'.
>
> (Kakar 1982: 23)

Yet the parallels between the two discourses are remarkable –

Kakar's chapter on the work of the pir shows the development of mutual admiration and understanding of overlapping discourses between the demonological and the psychological expert on mental illness.

Social, economic and gender context

Ann Phoenix (1988: 153) argues that analyses of class, race and gender are crucial to the understanding of any society, and of individual behaviours, 'since the intersection of these structural forces serves to locate individuals in their social positions and also to provide social construction of beliefs and identity'. In research on 'race' and health, the focus has been predominantly on a simplistic notion of minority cultures and not on the wider context of people's lives. I will offer two examples to illustrate the difficulty of isolating 'culture' from considerations of social-, economic- and gender-related factors.

The first example is from a qualitative study of working-class African-American mothers of children with sickle cell disease (SCD) by Shirley Hill (1994). Racism, deprivation and gender relations provide a strong, and necessary, backdrop for understanding the experiences of these mothers. They felt that poverty compromised their ability to make the home environment conducive to good care of a child with SCD. Racism was felt by many to be at the back of the lukewarm official response to SCD and the inadequate funding of screening and treatment programmes; women felt that SCD remains a low priority because it is a 'black disease', a sentiment also reported in British studies of SCD and thalassaemia (Anionwu 1993). Racial inequalities in the job market in America mean that few black men from poor areas find employment and consequently few are regarded by African-American women as marriageable. Most of the women were not married to the father of their child(ren) with SCD. They felt unable to influence the reproductive behaviour of their male partners; some fathers contested their paternity after mothers suggested that they may have sickle cell trait. In the absence of support from services and/or fathers of their children, most women relied on the strong system of kin-based informal support (largely from sisters and mothers). Hill makes a powerful observation on the mothers' choice to have children despite the risks of SCD. The powerful cultural ideology of motherhood served to undermine the power of medical education to effect change in repro-

ductive behaviour. According to Hill, mothers had three reproductive choices: to have partners tested; to have prenatal diagnosis and
selective abortion; or to forgo motherhood. However, in effect they
had little control or influence over their male partners, and services
for prenatal diagnosis were not always available.

To Hill:

> The only feasible option for most mothers who wanted to be sure
> not to pass the disease on to a child was to forgo motherhood,
> thus relinquishing one of the few areas of life over which they
> exercised control and from which they derived satisfaction. A
> diagnosis of SCD posed a threat to the reproductive autonomy
> of these mothers; they responded by denying, confounding, or
> doubting SCD medical knowledge, instead of accepting it.
>
> (Hill 1994: 72)

This wider contextualisation makes Hill's account a powerful one
and shows how the cultural norms and behaviours of these women are
inextricably interlinked with poverty, gender relations and racism.

My second example focuses on the hypothesis that consanguinity
causes the higher rates of congenital malformation and perinatal
mortality rates among babies of Pakistani-origin mothers and
shows the dangers of not taking into account socio-economic and
service-related factors in studying health and illness. Whereas in the
recent past higher perinatal mortality rates of Asian women have
been blamed on generalised cultural deviance, for the Pakistani women,
the focus now is on their high rates (around 50 per cent) of consanguineous marriages. In contrast, other personal (e.g., mothers' age, parity,
stature), service-related and socio-economic factors have received relatively little attention (Pearson 1991). I have argued elsewhere that
the research on consanguinity is of generally poor quality, suffers
from definitional problems (around what constitutes consanguinity
and ethnicity) and is usually based on selective and incomplete data
(Ahmad 1996). In particular, it fails to adequately address the
major confounding variables, such as social class and the quality of
general practitioner and maternity services, including the influence
of service providers, which may affect access to prenatal diagnosis
and selective terminations. The consanguinity hypothesis neatly
shifts the burden for poor birth outcome on to the victims. Currently, at least one health authority is translating this hypothesised
link into a health promotion campaign aimed at effecting change in
marriage patterns towards non-consanguineous marriages.

Cultural change

Like people in general, Britain's minority ethnic groups utilise a number of resources for cultural continuity: minority welfare and social institutions; religion; media; links with countries of origin; teaching of the mother tongue; literature, arts and music, for example. Often, encapsulation is enforced by outside hostility and 'sticking together' becomes an important tool for survival. However, cultural change is taking place for minority ethnic communities. Increased personal autonomy, less severe consequences of non-conformity, and social and structural changes are all important catalysts for change. For example, smaller houses have implications for the continuity of the traditional (though by no means universal) Asian extended family under one roof, and this may be exacerbated by the less localised job market for the second generation. Bhachu (1988) has noted the trend towards equalisation of power in gender relations in Sikh families as a consequence of women's involvement in the labour market. Change can also be externally imposed in terms of legal or social factors; for example, in the 1960s Sikh men often gave up their turbans and beards in view of the hostility from white people but later resisted legislation on the wearing of helmets for motorcyclists. These changes, however, are by no means evenly distributed.

Equally, cultural change and continuity are not absolutes. Neither is this necessarily peculiar to minority cultures; all cultures change over time (and at times suddenly, as in a revolution). Rao (1977: 21) notes, for example, that the assumption of a society or culture in a state of internal and external equilibrium is a fiction: 'In every living society, there is always some movement from within and some movement from without, and therefore there is always some change.' However, it may be that the pace of change in minority cultures in Britain may be more uneven, both for different constituencies (old, young, men, women, educated, etc.) within the same ethnic group and between different ethnic groups. Further, it may also lead to a greater disparity between cultural knowledge/beliefs and behaviour (Tripp-Reimer 1983; Modood, Beishon and Virdee 1994). This makes the notion of some unitary culture of particular ethnic groups or of a linear link between cultural beliefs and behaviour even more problematic.

I will offer an example of the complexity of disentangling continuity from change. Modood, Beishon and Virdee (1994) show differences in perspectives on marriage between Asian and African-Caribbean immigrants, and their children, the second generation, born or brought up in Britain. The first generation Asians regarded arranged marriage based on considerations of compatibility, of not just the couple but of the two families, as the only (and certainly the best) option and saw it as crucial to the survival of the extended family, carrying out familial obligations and care of the elderly and the sick. The second generation's views on marriage revolved around notions of romantic love, personal freedom and mutual compatibility. Although the second generation's views were not directly related to their choices – most had acceded or were willing to accede to their parents' wishes – the first generation recognised the need for greater say from their sons and daughters in their marriages than was the case for themselves. Other research confirms a process of negotiation and give and take between first and second generation in terms of retention of cultural values and beliefs (Drury 1991).

Considering the complexities of cultural change, describing the norms or predicting the behaviour of an ethnic group on the basis of cultural knowledge of the country of origin are impossible tasks. Phoenix (1988) describes the problems of explaining the behaviour of the British African-Caribbeans with reference to a simplistic notion of the culture of the Caribbean. First, it excludes black people from the category 'British'. The assumption is that the British have a distinct culture which can be defined in opposition to the Caribbean culture of the British African-Caribbeans (although in other discourses African-Caribbean cultures are regarded as impoverished versions of the British culture). Second, it oversimplifies the Caribbean culture as a unitary and static set of customs, beliefs, traditions and values when, in fact, the Caribbean is characterised by a diversity of identities, cultural traditions and ethnicities. Third, by promoting the conception of a homogenous Caribbean culture (and by implication a similarly undifferentiated British culture) it strengthens the assumption that all black people are different from all white people. Fourth, it equates culture with colour and fails to see culture as equally a product of gender, class or other power relations. Finally, it oversimplifies the notion of culture, ignoring its dynamism and diversity, its endurance as well as its malleability. For example, the culture of young black people in Britain builds on that of their parents and grandparents, as well as on the cultures of their white peers; it is a uniquely British construction. The points that

Phoenix makes are equally applicable to South Asian and other minority ethnic communities.

CULTURE AND HEALTH POLICY

Most of the early official interventions were aimed at effecting cultural change either in the service providers or, more often, in minority communities. Campaigns against surma and rickets are examples of this. The Stop Rickets Campaign, for example, recast the problem of vitamin D deficiency – acknowledged as a disease of poverty which was reduced in the white population with improvements in standards of living and housing, and interventions such as fortification of margarine with vitamin D and the universal availability of free milk to school children – in terms of cultural defects. Advice ranged from sunbathing and changes in diet and lifestyle to pronouncements that without Westernisation the Asians would never be able to rid themselves of their 'Asian' rickets (Ahmad 1989). Other initiatives included the production of texts for health care workers by Alex Henley at the National Extension College. In keeping with the emphasis on culture and difference, these texts concentrated on naming systems, dietary habits, religions, cultural beliefs, family structures, and so on (e.g. Henley 1979).

Perhaps the best-known intervention of the 1980s is the Asian Mother and Baby Campaign (AMBC). This was in many ways a continuation of the Stop Rickets Campaign, with funding from the same sources and the same senior management team. AMBC constructed problems of high perinatal mortality in terms of inadequate use of services; this was presumed to be located in the women's limited knowledge of services and their cultural values, and the health service providers' ignorance of these values, rather than in social class, racism or quality of care. Burden of change was largely placed on women. As Rocheron (1988) notes, the aim of AMBC was to accommodate rather than undermine professional practices. One way in which it differed from the earlier campaign on rickets was that there was, albeit belated, recognition of racism as an important factor in service delivery. This, however, was pushed on to the agenda by the experiences of the link workers, rather than being part of the campaign as originally conceived. Because of its neglect of structural issues and institutional racism – the link workers had a relatively low status and yet were expected to challenge the perspectives and practices of the people (nurses and doctors) to whom they were accountable – the campaign was heavily criticised by some Asian community groups as being 'racist' (Rocheron 1988). AMBC has led to some useful changes, however. For example, most of the participating health authorities retained link workers and, for some women at least, communication difficulties in English have eased. However, limited numbers and lack of adequate round-the-clock coverage still leave many Asian women to rely on crude sign language or family members (including children) when communicating with health professionals (Theodore-Gandi and Shaikh 1988). Equally, AMBC has not been able to challenge or change racially discriminatory practices.

An alternative approach aimed at providing advocacy support to women from minority ethnic groups has worked well in Hackney. Here, the 'advocates' are not located or accountable to NHS managers but to an independent agency. In an evaluation of the scheme, Parsons and Day (1992) suggest this as a progressive model of empowering women in their relationship with maternal health services. There is evidence that the scheme had a beneficial impact on birth outcome.

ANTI-RACISM AND HEALTH POLICY

Anti-racism in the health service is not a strong or long tradition. However, some initiatives are worth noting. First, and perhaps the most important site of struggles in the area of 'race' and health, are developments in the field of psychiatry. Here the radical critiques of the Black Health Workers and Patients' Group (1983), Mercer (1986), Fernando (1991) and Sashidharan and Francis (1993) Health are worth noting and have made an impact at the level of being recognised as important challenges to psychiatric orthodoxies. Radical alternatives to traditional psychiatric treatments have been proposed, including the Harambee Core and Cluster Project (Francis *et al.* 1988). The African-Caribbean Mental Health Association, under Francis, became a major dissenting voice in the 1980s and continues to function in that capacity. Focusing on the South Asian communities, the Confederation of Indian Organisations commissioned reviews of evidence on mental ill health and made policy suggestions (Beliappa 1991). Although these initiatives have not transformed the construction of minority ethnic communities' mental health problems or service delivery, they offer notable opposition to the dominant and often oppressive models of research and service delivery.

Second, whereas the rhetoric of specialist provision has been strong, the two particular conditions which predominantly affect minority ethnic communities, sickle cell disorders and thalassaemia, have only reluctantly been acknowledged by authorities. Considerable community action has been at the back of this limited official recognition. However, the change has been piecemeal and limited, services remain patchy and ill-co-ordinated, provision is service led, and patients with SCD and thalassaemia and their carers report unsympathetic and low-quality service support (Anionwu 1993; Davies, Modell and Wonke 1993).

Third, the 1988 report by the NAHA (National Association of Health Authorities), *Action Not Words*, highly critical of the lack of progress within the NHS, raised the profile of 'race' and health within health authorities. Although the report was itself criticised for not going far enough in locating inequalities in health and illness in their wider racialised context, its impact was felt across health authorities, at least in the short term. However, in the medium term, the resultant activity seems to have been largely at the level of public relations. Few if any authorities have devised policies to improve community involvement, needs assessment or service delivery. Effective equal opportunities policies are rare in the health care sector, and representation of minority ethnic communities on health authority and NHS trust boards remains very low. The recently established NHS Ethnic Health Unit, funded for three years from April 1994, has the task of affecting positive change in health provision through the purchasing mechanisms (Chan 1995). Despite having credible personnel and enjoying a strong degree of goodwill among black community groups and health workers, the unit's task seems beyond its resources and time-scale.

CONCLUDING COMMENTS

My main argument in this chapter is that common conceptions of 'culture' in research on the health and health care of minority ethnic communities lack a recognition of the dynamic and contextual nature of 'culture'. However, it is not just crude multiculturalism which has a trouble with culture. Crude anti-racism, in rejecting the multicultural orthodoxies, especially the neglect of structural and power relationships, also rejected 'culture' as an important element of the identity of racialised minorities. In the new construction of a wider, collective and political black identity cultural identities and resources, and their symbolic and practical significance was, to a large extent, sacrificed within some forms of anti-racism. Minority ethnic people became defined as the product of racisms they experienced. However, new forms of struggle around religious and cultural identity raised questions about the primacy of 'race' as the major or only form of identity, organisation and mobilisation. 'Culture' and its corollaries became recognised as legitimate and important aspects of ethnic identity and as resources for engagement with exclusionary discourses and practices. Although the dangers of absolutist notions of identity need to be avoided, a reappropriation of a much more politicised and contextual notion of 'culture' is a welcome development.

In studying health and illness among minority ethnic communities, the cultural context is of crucial importance. However, to be of value, either in explanatory or practical terms, 'culture' needs to be recognised as a context, itself flexible and contested, interacting with, shaping and shaped by other social and structural contexts of people's lives. Cultural norms, themselves contested and changing, represent flexible guidelines within which behaviour is negotiated rather than an 'independent variable' which is solely responsible for determining behaviour. Recognising this will be an important development in moving towards research on health and social care of minority ethnic communities which is of value for both its academic and practical contribution.

ACKNOWLEDGEMENTS

I am very grateful to Charles Husband, Charles Watters, my colleagues in the Social Policy Research Unit's 'race' and health care team and the editors for helpful criticism.

REFERENCES

Afshar, H. (1994) 'Muslim women in West Yorkshire: growing up with real and imaginary values amidst conflicting views of self and society' in H. Afshar and M. Maynard (eds) *The Dynamics of 'Race' and Gender: Some Feminist Interventions*. London: Taylor and Francis.

Ahmad, W. I. U. (1989) 'Policies, pills and political will: critique of policies to improve the health status of ethnic minorities', *Lancet* 1: 148–150.

Ahmad, W. I. U. (1992) 'The maligned healer: the "hakim" and western medicine', *New Community* 18(4): 521–536.

Ahmad, W. I. U. (1993) *'Race' and Health in Contemporary Britain*. Buckingham: Open University Press.

Ahmad, W. I. U. (1996) 'Consanguinity and related demons: science and racism in the debate on consanguinity and birth outcome' in S. Samson and N. South (eds) *Conflict and Consensus in Social Policy*. Basingstoke: Macmillan.

Ahmad, W. I. U., Baker, M. R. and Kernohan, E. E. M. (1991) 'General practitioners' perceptions of Asian patients', *Family Practice* 8(1): 52–56.

Ahmad, W. I. U., Kernohan, E. E. M. and Baker, M. R. (1989) 'Patients' choice of general practitioner: influence of patients' fluency in English and the ethnicity and sex of the doctor', *Journal of the Royal College of General Practitioners* 39: 153–155.

Ahmad, W. I. U. and Sheldon, T. (1993) '"Race" and statistics', in M. Hammersley (ed.) *Social Research: Philosophy, Politics and Practice*. London: Sage.

Ahmed, L. (1992) *Women and Gender in Islam: Historical Roots of a Modern Debate*. New Haven, CT and London: Yale University Press.

Alibhai-Brown, Y. (1993) 'Marriage of minds not hearts', *New Stateman and Society* 12/2: 28–29.

Anionwu, E. (1993) 'Sickle cell and thalassaemia: community experiences and official response', in W. I. U. Ahmad (ed.) *'Race' and Health in Contemporary Britain*. Buckingham: Open University Press

Balarajan, R., Yuen, P and Raleigh, V. (1989) 'Ethnic differences in general practitioner consultations', *British Medical Journal* 299: 958–960.

Barker, M. (1981) *The New Racism*. London: Junction Books.

Beliappa, J. (1991) *Illness or Distress? Alternative Models of Mental Health*. London: Confederation of Indian Organisations.

Bhachu, P. (1988) *'Apni marzi kardhi:* home and work: Sikh women in Britain' in S. Westwood and P. Bhachu (eds) *Enterprising Women: Ethnicity, Economy and Gender Relations*. London: Routledge.

Black Health Workers and Patients' Group (1983) 'Psychiatry and the corporate state', *Race and Class* 25(2): 49–64.

Bhopal, R. S. (1988) 'Health care for Asians: conflict in need, demand and provision' in Royal College of Physicians *Equity: A Pre-requisite for Health: Proceedings of the 1987 Summer Scientific Conference*. London: Royal College of Physicians.

Bhopal, R. S. and White, M. (1993) 'Health promotion for ethnic minorities: past, present and future' in W. I. U. Ahmad (ed.) *'Race' and Health in Contemporary Britain*. Buckingham: Open University Press.

Bowler, I. (1993) '"They're not the same as us"": midwives' stereotypes of South Asian women', *Sociology of Health and Illness* 15: 157–178.

Brah, A. (1992) 'Women of South Asian origin in Britain: issues and concerns' in P. Braham, A. Rattansi and R. Skellington (eds) *Racism and Antiracism: Inequalities, Opportunities and Policies*. London: Sage.

Carney, T. (1989) 'Ethnic population and general practitioner workload', *British Medical Journal* 299: 930–931.

Chan, M. (1995) 'The NHS Ethnic Health Unit', *Critical Public Health* 5(4): 41–46.

Crawford, R. (1977) 'You are dangerous to your health: the ideology and politics of victim blaming', *Internation Journal of Health Services* 7(4): 663–680.

Davies, S., Modell, B. and Wonke, B. (1993) 'The haemoglobinopathies: impact upon black and ethnic minority people', in A. Hopkins and V. Bahl (eds) *Access to Health Care for People from Black and Ethnic Minorities*. London: Royal College of Physicians.

Dodge, J. S. (ed.) (1969) *The Fieldworker in Immigrant Health*. London: Staples Press.

Dominelli, L. (1988) *Antiracist Social Work*. London: BASW/Macmillan

Donald, J. and Rattansi, A. (eds) (1992) *'Race', Culture and Difference*. London: Sage.

Drury, B. (1991) 'Sikh girls and the maintenance of an ethnic culture', *New Community* 17(3): 387–399.

Eade, J. (1989) *The Politics of Community*. Aldershot: Avebury.

Eade, J. (1995) 'The power of the experts: the plurality of beliefs and practices concerning health and illness among Bangladeshis', Roehampton Institute, London, unpublished manuscript.

Fernando, S. (1991) *Mental Health, Race and Culture*. Basingstoke: Macmillan/MIND.

Finch, J. (1989) *Family Obligations and Social Change*. Cambridge: Polity.

Francis, E., David, J., Johnson, N. and Sashidharan, S. (1988) 'Black people and psychiatry in the UK: an alternative to institutional care', *Psychiatric Bulletin* 13: 482–5.

Fuller, C. (1991) 'Kerala Christians and the caste system', in D. Gupta (ed.) *Social Stratification*. Oxford: Oxford University Press (Oxford in India Readings).

Gillam, S., Jarman, B., White, P. and Law, R. (1989) 'Ethnic differences in consultation rates in urban general practice', *British Medical Journal* 299: 953–957.

Healey, M. A. and Aslam, M. (1990) *The Asian Community: Medicines and Traditions*. Nottingham: Silver Link Publications.

Henley, A. (1979) *Asian Patients in Hospital and at Home*. London: Pitman Medical.

Hill, S. A. (1994) *Managing Sickle Cell Disease in Low Income Families*, Philadelphia, PA: Temple University Press.

Howitt, D. and Owusu-Bempah, J. (1994) *The Racism of Psychology: Time for Change*. Hemel Hempstead: Harvester Wheatsheaf.

Husband, C. (1991) ' "Race", conflictual politics and anti-racist social work: lessons from the past for action in the '90s' in Central Council for Education and Training in Social Work, *Anti-racist Social Work Education: Setting the Context for Change*. London: CCETSW.

Kakar, S. (1982) *Shamans, Mystics and Doctors: A Psychological Inquiry into India and Its Healing Traditions*. London: Unwin Hyman.

Kleinman, A. and Sung, L. H. (1979) 'Why do indigenous practitioners successfully heal?', *Social Science and Medicine* 13B: 7–26.

Kushnick, L. (1988) 'Racism, the National Health Service, and the health of black people', *International Journal of Health Services* 18(3): 457–470.

Lawrence, E. (1982) 'In the abundance of water the fool is thirsty: sociology and black pathology' in Centre for Contemporary Cultural Studies *The Empire Strikes Back*. London: Hutchinson.

McAvoy, B. R. and Raza, R. (1988) 'Asian women: (i) contraceptive knowledge, attitudes and usage, (ii) contraceptive services and cervical cytology', *Health Trends* 20: 11–17.

Mercer, K. (1986) 'Racism and transcultural psychiatry' in P. Miller and N. Rose (eds) *The Power of Psychiatry*. Cambridge: Polity Press.

Modood, T., Beishon, S. and Virdee, S. (1994) *Changing Ethnic Identities*. London: Policy Studies Institute.

NAHA (1988) *Action Not Words*, Birmingham: National Association of Health Authorities.

Nichter, M. (1980) 'The layperson's perception of medicine as perspective into the utilization of multiple therapy systems in the Indian context', *Social Science and Medicine* 14B: 225–233.

Parsons, L. and Day, S. (1992) 'Improving obstetric outcomes in ethnic minorities', *Journal of Public Health Medicine* 14: 183–192.

Pearson, M. (1986) 'Racist notions of ethnicity and culture in health education' in S. Rodmell and A. Watt (eds) *The Politics of Health Education*. London: Tavistock.

Pearson, M. (1991) 'Ethnic differences in health', *Archives of Disease in Childhood* 66: 88–90.

Phillimore, P. (1989) *Shortened Lives: Premature Death in North Tyneside*, Bristol Papers in Applied Social Studies 12.

Phoenix, A. (1988) 'Narrow definitions of culture: the case of early mother-hood', in S. Westwood and P. Bhachu (eds) *Enterprising Women: Ethnicity, Economy and Gender Relations*. London: Routledge.

Pillsbury, B. L. K. (1978) 'Doing the Month: confinement and convalescence of Chinese women after childbirth', *Social Science and Medicine* 12: 11–22.

Qureshi, B. (1989) *Transcultural Medicine*. Dundrecht: Kulwer Academic Publishers.

Rack, P. (1990) 'Psychological/psychiatric disorders' in B. R. McAvoy and L. J. Donaldson (eds) *Health Care for Asians*. Oxford: Oxford University Press.

Rao, V. K. R. V. (1977) 'Some thoughts on social change in India' in M. N. Srinivas, S. Seshaiah and V. S. Parthasarathy (eds) *Dimensions of Social Change in India*. New Delhi: Allied Publishers.

Research Unit in Health and Behavioural Change (RUHBC) (1989) *Changing the Public Health*. Chichester: John Wiley.

Rocheron, Y. (1988) 'The Asian Mother and Baby Campaign: the construction of ethnic minority health needs', *Critical Social Policy* 22: 4–23.

Sashidharan, S. and Francis, E. (1993) 'Epidemiology, ethnicity and schizophrenia' in W. I. U. Ahmad (1993) *'Race' and Health in Contemporary Britain*. Buckingham: Open University Press.

Sheldon, T. and Parker, H. (1992) 'The use of "ethnicity" and "race" in health research: a cautionary note' in W. I. U. Ahmad (ed.) *The Politics of 'Race' and Health*. Bradford: Race Relations Research Unit, University of Bradford.

Sivanandan, A. (1991) 'Black struggles against racism' in Central Council for Education and Training in Social Work *Anti-racist Social Work Education: Setting the Context for Change*. London: CCETSW.

Theodore-Gandi, B. and Shaikh, K. (1988) *Maternity Services Consumer Survey*. Bradford: Bradford Health Authority.

Thomas (1992) 'Religion and ageing in the Indian tradition', *Ageing and Society* 12: 105–113.

Tripp-Reimer, T. (1983) 'Retention of folk-healing practice (*matiasma*) among four generations of Urban Greek immigrants', *Nursing Research* 32(2): 97–101.

Watson, J. L. (1977) *Between Two Cultures: Migrants and Minorities in Britain*. Oxford: Blackwell.

Watters, C. (1996) 'Representations and realities: black people, community care and mental illness' in W. I. U. Ahmad and K. Atkin (eds) *'Race' and Community Care*. Buckingham: Open University Press.

Williams, F. (1989) *Social Policy: A Critical Introduction*. Cambridge: Policy Pess

Williams F (1996) ' "Race" welfare and community care: a historical perspective' in W. I. U. Ahmad and K. Atkin (eds) *'Race' and Community Care*. Buckingham: Open University Press.

Wright, C. (1983) 'Language and communication problems in the Asian community', *Journal of the Royal College of General Practitioners* 33: 1–4.

Chapter 10

'How should I live?'
Bangladeshi people and non-insulin-dependent diabetes

David Kelleher and Sharif Islam

INTRODUCTION

Diabetes is a condition which is caused by the failure of the body to produce sufficient insulin to convert food eaten into energy. In the case of children or other people who develop what is known as 'insulin-dependent diabetes', the symptoms are likely to be weight loss, extreme thirst and a need to urinate frequently. Their condition may deteriorate rapidly. In many cases with older people who develop what is known as 'non-insulin-dependent diabetes' the disease is asymtomatic but its presence may be indicated by the person needing to drink excessive quantities of liquid and urinating frequently. Tiredness is also likely to be a symptom. It affects about 2 per cent of the population of England and about 70 per cent of these will have the non-insulin-dependent type of diabetes. Like many chronic illnesses, diabetes has to be managed by the patients themselves in the contexts of their everyday lives. For people with non-insulin-dependent diabetes this means controlling what they eat and, for many, taking tablets to aid the production of insulin. They are also encouraged to take exercise and to avoid becoming obese. Many diabetic people do not find this easy (Kelleher 1988) as they have other concerns in their lives which often claim priority, in their view, over managing their diabetes. Some people find it difficult to control their eating and tablet-taking because of their work situation while others find that it is difficult to eat the kind of healthy foods recommended by doctors and nurses because of the preferences of other family members. All diabetic people have to weigh up these concerns in the process of integrating the diabetic treatment regimen with the other structures of relevance (Schutz 1971) which normally shape their everyday lives.

It has been noticed that in a number of South Asian populations living in England there is a much higher prevalence of non-insulin-dependent diabetes compared with the overall population of England (Mather and Keen 1985). McKeigue et al. (1988) have estimated that in the Bangladeshi population living in East London the prevalence is three times as high as in the white population. It also appears that Bangladeshi people are developing diabetes at younger ages than the white English population. Epidemiological research has not been able to positively identify any single dietary item which might explain the differences in prevalence rates. A number of other hypotheses have been put forward, including the rather speculative 'thrifty gene hypothesis' (McKeigue, Shah and Marmot 1991). This suggests that the people who were most likely to survive in countries where there have been periodic crop failures and famines were people who were predisposed to put on fat around the stomach. They were then able to utilise this in a period of famine. Now, living in conditions of comparative abundance, it is said that the predisposition to obesity is likely to lead to the development of non-insulin-dependent diabetes. While the search for both the cause of diabetes and the variations in rates between different populations and ethnic groups (Dowse et al. 1990) goes on, the problems of living with diabetes remain. It seemed important, therefore, to try to find out how Bangladeshi people were managing their diabetes. The results of the study reported here suggest that Bangladeshi people have additional structures of relevance which guide them in the way they go about the process of integrating the treatment regimen with their everyday activities. Principally, these other structures of relevance come from their Bangladeshi culture and from their Muslim beliefs and practices, and it is these which are described in this chapter. It is important to emphasise here that many diabetic people, not just Bangladeshi people, find difficulties in integrating the treatment regimen into their everyday lives and that what is sometimes referred to as 'non-compliance' is common. The view taken here is that non-compliance is less often a case of wilful neglect and more often the result of people struggling to integrate the varying structures of relevance in their lives with the medical treatment regimen. This is not to say that all Bangladeshi people have the same priorities; I am not arguing that they behave like Garfinkel's 'cultural dopes' (Garfinkel 1967) who do not have to interpret situations for themselves. It is not the case that all Bangladeshi people's behaviour can be understood simply by knowing their culture in a generalised way, but rather that they may share the same structures of relevance, the same ideas of what is important, but they draw on their culture in different ways in constructing explanatory models (Kleinman 1980) to use in shaping their everyday lives with diabetes.

METHODOLOGY

Most of the Bangladeshi people living in the Tower Hamlets district of East London come from the villages of Sylhet district. According to the 1991 census data the majority of this Bangladeshi community live in either local authority housing or housing association property. Two-thirds of households do not have a car, over one-third of the economically active people are unemployed and one-third of the households include in them someone who has a limiting long-standing illness. It is also a very young population, with over half under 20. It is a poor community. Jones states that 'the statistical data available almost certainly understate the extent of disadvantage experienced by ethnic minorities' (Jones 1993: 149). He adds that this is particularly likely to be true in the case of the Bangladeshi people.

The sample of 40 non-insulin-dependent people in this study, 25 men and 15 women appeared to be representative of the sample population. Only four of the men were working and one was a student. None of the women worked outside of the home. A quarter of the sample could not read and write in Bengali and only three could read and write in English. A quota sample was used to achieve a sample with a range of age groups, but in some cases some of the older men were not certain of their age. This is not surprising, as it is more common to celebrate on the anniversaries of people's deaths rather than on their birthdays in Bangladeshi culture.

The interviews were carried out in the Sylheti dialect by Sharif Islam and took place in the respondents' homes, apart from one interview which was conducted at the business premises of the respondent. The fact that Sharif was a man interviewing women did not appear to be a problem, although in some cases the respondent had invited another woman friend to be present, and in one case a husband took time off from work so that he could be present for the interview. Thirty other family members, wives, daughters and some husbands were also interviewed to collect additional data on how the diabetic person was managing their diabetes. The interviews with respondents lasted for about one and a half hours and the interview data was supplemented by other data collected by Sharif Islam, who lives in the community. On some occasions respondents appeared puzzled by the fact that Sharif Islam was asking them questions about their culture when he himself was a member of their community, an insider. Another method was therefore tried, with Kelleher asking the questions and Islam acting as an interpreter. This was successful in some ways, as people found it more understandable that an outsider should be asking such questions, but there were occasions when people appeared reluctant to say, in front of an outsider, anything which seemed to reflect badly on themselves or their community. After one interview the respondent said to Sharif Islam in Bengali:

> But the problem is you were recording so I felt extra burden to talk to him [DK] about our religion. Because if I say something wrong he will misjudge our whole community.
>
> (no. 38)

We were welcomed in every home and on almost all occasions we were offered tea and biscuits; in one home we were offered tea and biscuits only to be told a few minutes later that they had no tea left. In one or two homes Sharif Islam stayed for a meal and got drawn into helping children with homework. Some of the interviews gave the opportunity for participant observation and were far from being the formal type of interaction described in textbooks on methods, as some notes made at the time of one interview make clear.

> The father of eight children (the diabetic person). All the children are in the house, one is clinging to his father and another is sitting on his knee for most of the interview. His wife brought tea and biscotte type toast for us but the family did not share it with us. She said nothing although she stayed in the room the whole time. There was a sofa, one armchair and a white wooden chair and a small coffee table with one leg missing, as we discovered when we put the tape recorder on it. There was a television set and on the walls some holy pictures but there did not appear to be a prayer corner. There was a smell of nappies in the room. The children seemed quite lively and were interested in us.

Another interview took place in an office workshop above a Bangladeshi video and tape shop, and the music from there came wafting up during the interview. The office was up a rickety flight of wooden stairs and it was full of patterns of leather clothes. An old man worked in a corner cutting out leather. The insider status of Sharif Islam was essential in getting access to these respondents and in gaining their trust, and was necessary when it came to translating the interviews and interpreting the data, but it should be recognised that attempting to be an observing stranger asking naive questions about common-sense assumptions and at the same time passing as one of the group is difficult to achieve in practice.

The interviews were tape recorded and translated into English. The analysis was carried out by constructing a summary of responses to particular topics and then identifying themes in the data. The themes that will be discussed are grounded in the data.

THEMES FROM THE DATA

One of the topics that we asked questions about was the food people ate. Controlling eating is a key part of the diabetes treatment regimen but, because eating is as much concerned with social relationships as it is with providing energy, it is as important to find out why people eat as it is to know what they eat. Health professionals do not always seem to recognise this, as a short report of a study by Peterson et al. indicates (Peterson *et al.* 1986). They claim that their study was the first detailed study of the diets of 'Asian' diabetics in this country, and after describing the kinds and amounts of foods eaten by the people in the study they conclude that:

> There is a pressing need for culturally acceptable educational aids that recognise the regional differences between 'Asian' communities. Such aids should encourage a reduced consumption of refined carbohydrates and saturated fats and an increased consumption of unrefined carbohydrates rich in fibre.
>
> (Peterson *et al.* 1986: 171–172)

The Bangladeshi people in this study ate traditional foods in most cases, with rice, vegetables, fish and mutton being the main ingredients. These were generally eaten in curries. Chapattis were also eaten and some still ate *mistee*, Bangladeshi sweets. Other foods such as rice crispies, biscuits and bread had been added to the traditional ones, and the milk which was used had often been boiled, which made it taste like the sweetened evaporated kind of milk. Most of the people also had *pan*, the betel-nut leaf which is filled with a variety of substances including tobacco and is chewed by both men and women.

As would be expected, the people in the study expressed a range of views about their diet but most were making some attempt to control what they had to eat, generally by having less sugar and less rice and weaker curries as well as by trying to avoid rich foods at wedding parties and other celebrations. Everyone said that they found it very difficult to reduce the amount of rice that they ate and some complained that the amount of food they were supposed to eat was too little, 'only enough for a chicken', and the lack of food made them feel weak. One woman of 35, when asked what she had to eat during the Eid (festival day after Ramadan) said:

All the traditional pies, cakes, puddings, pillau rice, meat, curry.

(no. 6)

Others were much stricter in what they accepted. A man of 62 said:

Recently I was invited to several marriage parties. I told them directly 'I can go if you arrange fish and brown rice for me'.

(no. 16)

A related theme to describing what their meals consisted of was identifying their attitudes to food and fasting. It is clear that food is important in a number of ways. In all societies it plays a part in social relationships for both men and women; to accept food from someone is a sign of friendship and to refuse it would be interpreted as a withdrawal of friendship, but in this Bangladeshi community food seemed to have a greater significance than it does in a white English community. The exchange of food and sweets plays a part in the celebrations around religious events such as Shab-e-borat, when God is said to be weighing people's past deeds and deciding their fates. There is also Kurbani, a time when an animal such as a sheep is given for sacrifice and one third of it is given to relatives and another third to the poor. It is therefore not always easy to refuse food. A man in his fifties spoke about what he did when he was offered food by friends or relatives:

I don't eat anything there. Sometimes for formality I eat a little bit just to save their face.

(no. 17)

A woman of similar age said:

> I drink tea without sugar. About biscuits, even if it is sweet I
> have one or two for courtesy, just to save face.
>
> (no. 1)

One of the well-educated people, who was also one of the few who
was working, explained that:

> In any Bangladeshi function, may be religious occasion or a
> social occasion or a cultural programme or any get-together it is
> a must to have sweets.
>
> (no. 31)

There is therefore a social pressure to offer and accept food which
can make it difficult to keep to a medically prescribed diet. There is
also the feeling, that many other lay people besides Bangladeshi
people have, that food is essentially good for you and to deny yourself food is unnatural. All of them remembered being told by the
doctors that sugar was bad for them, but some felt that it was still
necessary to have some. A woman said:

> If there is no salt and sugar in a person he gets down [weak].
> That's why I take some sugar.
>
> (no. 36)

It was also noticeable that when we were offered tea Kelleher was
asked whether he took sugar but it was assumed that Islam would.
Food was seen as an important part of social life but was also seen as
something to be enjoyed as part of the good life. And one man said:

> Now Mister, you are a human being. I am a human being. We
> are all descendants of Adam. If I don't eat what my soul wants it
> is like killing myself in other way.
>
> (no. 4)

People often talked about rice as being 'soul food' and about
themselves as being 'rice-eating people'. A young wife of a diabetic
man whose registered age was 58 but whom she said was 80 said
that although, she controlled his food, she gave him:

> the things his soul wants to eat.
>
> (no. 10)

The significance attached to rice in the Bangladeshi culture is
considerable. This is no doubt partly because it is traditional and

reminds people of their home country and also because of the traditional ritual of introducing babies to rice by touching their lips with a grain of rice in a simple ceremony when they are about 6-months-old. At this ceremony (Annyaprashon) the adults eat sweet rice as rice puddings (*firni*). Although rice is a traditional and central part of Bangladeshi culture, there does not appear to be any religious imperative to eat it, however, and the reference to 'soul food' appears to mean no more than it is something which gives great satisfaction and reminds them their of their homeland:

> If I eat chapatti for my diet I will not be content but if I eat same amount of rice I will be.
>
> (no. 27)

There is a wide range of cultural influences which people may consider in the process of settling on a diet which takes account of medical advice by attempting to integrate it into their existing and developing lay knowledge. Many expressed the view that vegetables which came from under the ground were not good for people with diabetes. There is also the belief that green, unripe fruits are good and that anything bitter is also good and acts to counteract the sugar which diabetic people cannot deal with. There are ideas about keeping the blood in balance and certain things like cumin seeds are seen as good for diabetes but inclined to make the body dry inside. There are also issues around sour things, with some seeing them as foods that are specially liked by young women, but others saying that sour things are bad for diabetes:

> Sour things are bad. If I eat a thing called Satkara [a plant of the citrus variety whch is a popular ingredient in curries] . . . that one will pull up your diabetes the moment after you eat it.
>
> (no. 23)

Karella, a bitter vegetable, was widely used, with some saying that they fried it and others that they drank the bitter juice. Some said that they had been told by their doctor to use karella, and one person claimed that it was on the hospital diet sheet, which is an interesting example of doctors being prepared to work with lay ideas. There is some evidence (Bailey, Day and Leatherdale 1986) that karella does help to lower blood sugar levels which has, no doubt, helped to persuade doctors to accept it.

As well these traditional ideas which people draw on or are aware of in developing their ways of managing diabetes there are the new ideas which they may get from their children or from television. Although traditionally, plump people have been considered to be healthy and good-looking in Bangladeshi culture, there is a growing awareness that slimness is more healthy and it is coming to be seen as more attractive. One young woman was watching an exercise programme on afternoon television when we went to interview her. She was aged 34 and said she had bought slimming foods:

> I want to become slim. I tried many things. I controlled my foods and many other ways. None was effective. I worry about it because I want a slim body.

> (no. 28)

While she was unusual amongst the people we interviewed, in her desire to be slim and in her willingness to try slimming foods she may have been more typical of a younger generation than the majority of those who were interviewed. There were a number of parents, for example, who said that their children wanted to eat chips, fish fingers, rice crispies and chocolate. There was a very exceptional man who said that he and his wife had taken their daughter for a treat to McDonalds even though they realised that the food was not halal. There are arguments in the community about the acceptability of such food, and some are prepared to see it as mokru, food which is neither halal nor haram. Because it is not halal, food which is mokru can be eaten, but after eating it it is necessary to carry out a washing ritual before engaging in prayer.

As well as attempting to integrate the medical regimen with traditional Bangladeshi ideas about eating and food these people were therefore also attempting to choose Western foods which they and their children could eat without contravening their beliefs and without having too many arguments about food. A number of mothers, like mothers in any cultural group, were worried that their children did not want to eat proper food, only crisps, sweets and cola, but for some it was also a question of bringing them up as Bangladeshi children; food played a part in maintaining a sense of identity:

> They don't like to eat our foods all the times. They try to eat this country's foods all the time. But I insist them to eat our foods otherwise they wouldn't grow healthy. Moreover, they need to learn our culture.

> (no. 18)

As well as integrating Western foods into their eating they were all making some attempt to incorporate medical advice into their eating patterns, mainly by reducing the amount of sugar and sweets and by reducing the amount of rice, by eating brown rice instead of white rice, which meant cooking it separately from the rest of the family, and by having weaker curries. Some found it hard:

Brown rice is hard. I get problem to swallow it, they hurt my neck. I get choked so I have decided to go back to white rice.

(no. 23)

This man said that he would not tell his doctor that he was doing it, though. Another man who seemed to be managing well said that in hospital they had tried to give him special diabetic cream, but he had refused and told them:

If I control diabetes my way I feel better

(no. 25)

Another man who was making a determined effort to follow medical advice said that he was eating less than the dietician recommended. The diet sheet said that he could eat one banana a day but he did not eat any. He had also given up grapes and sugar and biscuits and had one apple a fortnight instead of one a day. He had changed to brown bread and brown rice and his wife made curries less spicy for him.

Although many people did not have a good understanding of the medical view of diabetes, they did generally accept the link between eating and controlling the level of sugar in the blood, although they sometimes were confused by the fact that they might have a raised level of sugar according to a urine test but not according to a blood test. One woman who said that the doctors had proved that she had diabetes said:

Diabetes hasn't got into my blood yet, only in urine.

(no. 28)

On the whole, they saw their diabetes as a problem which had to be managed medically; they did not appear to think that forest or folk medicines had much to offer them, apart from the widely used karella. Neither did they think that the wearing of amulets had much power to control diabetes, although some thought that they were useful for things like stomach pains and for some 'external' (psychological) illness, illnesses which 'come from above'.

The difficulties described so far have been seen as the result of people trying to integrate the traditional cultural ideas about food with the ideas that they are taking up from the global, rice-crispie culture and prescribed medical diets. Apart from the broadly based cultural ideas it was clear that many were strongly influenced in deciding what they could eat by the beliefs of their Muslim religion and it is this influence which will now be described.

The most powerful concern was the need to eat only food which was halal, and this included avoiding foods which had in them fats from animals which had not been ritually slaughtered as well as not eating pork. Foods which are haram were avoided, and although no one said that they did eat foods such as shrimps or crabs, one respondent explained that these were traditionally categorised as mokru, not able to be clearly categorised, and although they could be eaten it would be necessary to perform ritual cleaning afterwards before going to the mosque. Although people varied in how strictly they followed this halal rule there was only one person who was prepared to disregard it; for everyone else it was an important concern and for some it was clearly more important than following a medical regimen.

One man who was very concerned to eat only halal food said that he did not eat beef because it often comes from English slaughterhouses which are not halal. He also said that when he first came to England it was not always as easy as it is now to get halal meat, so that he and the other men that he was living with would slaughter a chicken in the bathroom to ensure that it was halal. He said:

> Obviously haram things are bad for health. That is why our prophet told us not to eat haram things.
>
> (no. 37)

Another man who was trying to control his diabetes by eating green mangoes and karella, but who was also one of the few who were doing urine or blood tests, said that haram food was bad for health and took care to buy only halal food, including bread and biscuits. He said that:

> I am a Mohammadi [follower of the prophet Mohammed]. . . . If I eat something not halal I will have to vomit or I will have diarrhoea.
>
> (no. 29)

Some of those who took care to buy only food which was halal, including bread and biscuits, said that the Young Muslim Organisation had produced a list of ingredients which had to be avoided. Others took a more relaxed view and said that they did not eat haram meat but did not bother when it came to bread and biscuits. As one said:

> I normally eat Mother's Pride. They said it is halal and I believe and take it.
>
> (no. 34)

One expressed the view that there are many important things which a good Muslim should do but:

> instead we fuss about useless things
>
> (no. 28)

Another aspect of being a Muslim is the requirement to fast at Ramadan, and this could be seen as something which might be problematic for people who are controlling a chronic illness by regulating their eating. In fact, the great majority of people did fast for the month of Ramadan. Of the three who said that they did not fast, one was a woman who had recently had a baby and so was excused fasting for 40 days. Only a few of the remaining 37 said that this made it difficult to control their diabetes. One (no. 34) said that his diabetes got upset in Ramadan and he could not keep it under control. Another complained that when he is fasting:

> I feel weak. My head spins but we [Muslims] can't avoid fasting. Being a Muslim we have to fast. It is God's order.
>
> (no. 29)

Another person interpreted the rule differently. Although she was a firm believer and said that she could not eat without saying a prayer, she had given up her fast because, she said:

> We have clear instruction from God that we can stop fasting and other practices if our health is in danger. Also I was told by the doctor.
>
> (no. 33)

It is interesting to note that the authority of the doctor came second to the authority of God, indicating that for this person, at least, the medical rules are likely to be considered secondary in the process of integrating them with rules derived from being a Muslim. This was further illustrated by the fact that, for some, fasting also meant that they did not take their tablets. One woman in her thirties admitted that she did not tell the diabetic liaison nurse that she was going to fast:

> I thought that if I tell them they would mind. They wouldn't come and see me . . . I have diabetes but if I disobey God's order something worse can happen to me. We are Muslim – they do not understand what is good and bad for us.
>
> (no. 18)

Many of them said that they actually felt better when they were fasting and attributed this to the fact that fasting is God's work and therefore God looks after them. Some admitted that they had problems after Ramadan, though.

Kleinman suggests (1980) that people develop their own explanatory models from a matrix containing several levels, including the individual's experience, the family's knowledge and the beliefs in the culture of the community. The evidence from this study is that the Bangladeshi people in this sample did make use of their own experience and also drew on cultural beliefs about food, such as that vegetables from under the ground are not good for them, that curries should not be too strong for sick people and that bitter things are good because the bitterness counteracts the sweetness which, as diabetic, people they cannot deal with. They were also acquiring some knowledge from the medical people with whom they came into contact. The most powerful influence on their daily lives, though, on their eating and on the way they managed their diabetes, was undoubtably their Muslim religion. Although not everyone interpreted the teachings of the Qur'ān in the same way, and indeed many of them could not read it, it was something which provided them with many practical rules for living in a much more direct way than the Christian religion does.

Their culture and in particular their religion gave them a sense of identity and of belonging to a community in an environment which was strange, unfriendly and sometimes hostile to the extent that husbands and parents generally were quite often fearful for their children. They saw themselves as Bangladeshis and, to varying degrees, Muslims, and frequently talked about 'our people'. In many ways the problems they experienced in integrating the medical understanding of diabetes with the cultural beliefs and religious rules were an example of the larger problem they faced, a problem which was only partly about what they could and could not eat and was really about two different styles of thinking about life. What they were having to adjust to was the difference between living in a traditional society where behaviour is largely governed by customs and rules, and where problems are managed by faith, ritual and trust in God, where questions of life and death are answered by consulting the holy texts and, on the other hand, being confronted by a problem defined by modern medicine, which has to be managed by measuring the level of sugar in their urine and by calculating how much they should eat. Many of them recognised that the tablets they took and the food they ate had an effect on how they felt, the level of symptoms they experienced, and some of them made determined efforts to carry out the instructions of the dietitian and the doctor; but many of them seemed to be doing so to relieve the symptoms and partly to avoid having to move on to what they saw as a more serious stage of diabetes, that is, having to inject themselves with insulin. The fear of injections motivated their compliance. Very few people mentioned what are usually called the complications of diabetes, such as loss of eyesight, kidney damage, loss of toes or limbs as a result of neuropathy and the consequent need for amputation, although one man said that:

> Diabetes causes weakness, it takes away people's eyesight, it takes away people's sex power.
>
> (no. 23)

It seemed that very often people were attempting to reconcile in an *ad hoc* way one rule with another rule rather than engaging in the kind of rational calculation that modern medicine expects diabetic patients to engage in, not just to reduce the level of symptoms but in order to prevent premature death from the complications of diabetes. Although some people made statements such as 'I have faith in my doctor' and 'You can't disbelieve the doctors, can you?', it was much more common to hear people say 'Allah has given me this problem' and 'It is God's order so I got diabetes' or 'Everything is God's play'. That they were experiencing difficulties in attempting to integrate the kinds of knowledge was sometimes shown during the course of one interview as one man said first:

> Diet is the most important thing to control diabetes.

And later:

> You know a few days ago someone told me fenugreek is good for diabetes. I instantly bought it. Why shouldn't I give it a try? It is

an illness so there must be a remedy. Maybe fenugreek, who knows?

He also said:

> I believe in what is said in the Qur'ān. Djinns and other supernatural powers exist. I also believe in God, so I believe in Fate.
>
> (no. 8)

The idea that they should control their blood sugar level in order to reduce the risk of premature death was not mentioned by anyone. There was an assumption that how long they would live was ultimately in the hands of God:

> God has written how long I am going to live in his book. He will decide when I should die. It is upon Him.
>
> (no. 3)

The idea of changing their lifestyle in order to reduce the risk of developing the complications was not a way of thinking that was familiar to many of the people in this study. Their attitude to life and death was that of people used to living in a traditional society where there is a trust in the future, whereas in a modern one the future is uncertain and the idea of changing your lifestyle to reduce a risk is a way of attempting to get a fix on the future, an essentially a modern way of thinking as Giddens suggests:

> Modernity is essentially a Post-traditional order. The transformations of time and space, coupled with the disembedding mechanisms, propel social life away from the hold of pre-established precepts or practices.
>
> (Giddens 1991: 20)

The problem that these Bangladeshi people were facing was much more than simply making personal choices about what to eat. Although that in itself was a problem, because in Bangladeshi society food appears to carry many symbolic meanings and they were more used to deciding what to eat by reference to custom and the rules relating to the halal/haram distinction than by personal choices developed in a world where different types of food are constantly being advertised and displayed. As well as being confronted by this, 'the dialectic of the local and the global' (Giddens 1991: 22) in integrating their traditional foods and choosing new, internationally available foods like rice crispies, fish fingers and crisps and a variety of different kinds of bread and biscuits, their · traditional ways of thinking about life and death were being challenged by a medical treatment which is predicated on a notion of risk reduction and involves a radically different form of thinking from that which is common in traditional societies. The question 'How should I live?' was not a question they asked themselves, but it is a question that people in modern societies have to ask themselves as they struggle to make sense of the weight of advice they are given by health professionals. Another way of conceptualising it is to see the difference between the types of society as Durkheim described them:

> If when we are sick we take the care of ourselves following the doctor's orders, it is not only out of respect for his authority but also because we hope that we will be cured ... It is a utilitarian consideration... It is quite otherwise with moral rules... it is necessary for us to yield not in order to avoid disagreeable results... but very simply because we must, regardless of the consequences our conduct may have for us.
>
> (Durkheim 1972: 98–99)

For many of the people in this study the risk they recognised, but did not have to calculate, was the risk of eating something which was not halal, a risk of breaking a moral law; but if that did happen they appeared to feel that if they did it unknowingly it was not their fault but the fault of the person who sold it to them. If they later learnt that they had eaten something which was not Halal there was always a prayer which could be said.

CONCLUSION

This study has attempted to describe the social reality of the 40 people with diabetes who were all in the process of finding their individual ways of managing their condition. Some of them were testing their blood sugar levels and making adjustments to what they ate in order to achieve control, others were relying on eating more karella while some were just trying to eat less rice, eat brown rice, eat weaker curries. They were trying to follow the medical advice as they remembered it. Changing eating patterns is not easy, as thousands of people trying to slim will testify, but it is apparent from what people said that, for these Bangladeshi people, changing what they ate was not simply a question of changing their personal preferences; what they ate had a symbolic significance because of the links that their food had with their identity as rice-eating Bangladeshis and with the strong Muslim influence on their identity. Even one man who said he paid little attention to the halal/haram distinction described himself as a Muslim and said:

> I wouldn't say that it [rice] is a soul food but it is something you are brought up with and something that psychologically affects us.
>
> (no. 27)

Their cultural identity as Bangladeshis and Muslims were important structures of relevance in their lives which gave them a sense of priorities as they sought to incorporate the medical regimen of being a diabetic person into their daily existence in a developing culture. As the variety of quotes show, some individuals placed more importance on what they took to be the rules of their religion than others; some gave priority to the traditional ways they had grown up with and there were signs that a few were giving priority to adapting their lifestyle so that they and their children took some things from the non-Muslim world around them.

All of them, within the material constraints of their situations, were actively constructing their lives as people with diabetes and their cultural beliefs were one of the resources they used. The clear message of the study is that there is not one stereotypical Bangladeshi identity; they are not, to use Garfinkel's phrase again, 'cultural dopes' who can be understood without listening to their individual accounts. The frameworks, the structures of relevance that they draw on are shared, but they individually construct their lives within them. If health professionals want to help them in the process of integrating the medical treatment regimen into their lives, they need to learn to listen and to create the kind of relationship in which patients feel that they can say that they want to fast and can ask for advice about whether they need to take their medication. God may remain in front but the doctor may then not be far behind.

ACKNOWLEDGEMENTS

We would like to thank Shamsul Alam for his helpful comments on an earlier draft of this chapter.

This research was funded by the British Diabetic Association but the conclusions drawn are those of the authors and are not necessarily shared by the Association.

REFERENCES

Bailey, C., Day, C. and Leatherdale, B. (1986) 'Traditional treatments for diabetes from Asia and the West Indies', *Practical Diabetes* 3(4): 190–192.

Dowse, G., Gareebooh, N., Zimmet, P. Alberti, K., Tuomilehto, J., Fareed, D., Brissomette, L. and Finch, C. (1990) *Diabetes* 39(3): 309–316.

Durkheim, E. (1972) *Selected Writings* (ed. A. Giddens). Cambridge: Cambridge University Press.

Garfinkel, H. (1967) *Studies in Ethnomethodology*. Cambridge: Polity Press.

Giddens, A. (1991) *Modernity and Self-identity*. Cambridge: Polity Press.

Jones, T. (1993) *Britain's Ethnic Minorities*. London: Policy Studies Institute.

Kelleher, D. (1988) 'Coming to terms with diabetes: coping strategies and non-compliance' in R. Anderson and M. Bury *Living with Chronic Illness*. London: Allen and Unwin.

Kleinman, A. (1980) *Patients and Healers in the Context of Culture*. Berkeley, CA: University of California Press.

McKeigue, P., Marmot, M., Court, Y., Cottier, D., Rahman, S. and Riemersma, R. (1988) 'Diabetes, hyperinsulinaemia and coronary risk factors in Bangladeshis in East London,' *British Heart Journal* 60: 390–396.

McKeigue, P., Shah, B. and Marmot, M. (1991) 'Relation of central obesity and insulin resistance with high diabetes prevalence and cardio-vascular risk in South Asians', *Lancet* 337: 382–386.

Mather, H. and Keen, H. (1985) 'The Southall diabetes survey: prevalence of known diabetes in Asians and Europeans', *British Medical Journal* 291: 1081–1094.

Peterson, D., Dattani, J., Baylis, J. and Jepson, E. (1986) 'Dietary practices of Asian diabetics', *British Medical Journal* 292: 170–171.

Ramaiya, K., Kodala, V. and Alberti, K. (1990) 'Epidemiology of diabetes in Asians of the sub-continent', *Diabetes Metabolism Review* 6(3): 125–146.

Schutz, A. (1971) *Collected Papers* (vol. 2). The Hague: Martinus Nijhof.

Index